Steps on the Road to Medicare

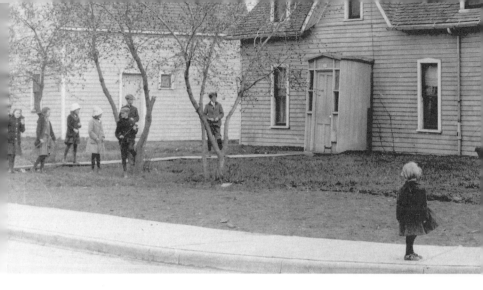

STEPS ON THE ROAD
TO MEDICARE

Why Saskatchewan Led the Way

C. Stuart Houston

McGill-Queen's University Press

Montreal & Kingston • London • Ithaca

© McGill-Queen's University Press, 2002
ISBN 0-7735-2366-9 (cloth)
ISBN 0-7735-2550-5 (paper)

Legal deposit fourth quarter 2002
Bibliothèque nationale du Québec

Printed in Canada on acid-free paper that is 100% ancient forest free
(100% post-consumer recycled), processed chlorine free.

Funding for this book has been received from the University of Saskatchewan
through its Publication Fund.

McGill-Queen's University Press acknowledges the support of the Canada
Council for the Arts for our publishing program. We also acknowledge the
financial support of the Government of Canada through the Book Publishing
Industry Development Program (BPIDP) for our publishing activities.

National Library of Canada Cataloguing in Publication Data

Houston, C. Stuart (Clarence Stuart), 1927–
    Steps on the road to medicare : why Saskatchewan led the way / C. Stuart
Houston.

Includes bibliographical references and index.
ISBN 0-7735-2366-9 (bnd)
ISBN 0-7735-2550-5 (pbk)

1. Medical care – Saskatchewan – History. 2. Medical policy – Saskatchewan –
History. 3. Health care reform – Saskatchewan – History. I. Title.

RA412.5C3H67 2002   362.1'097124   C2002-904008-6

This book was designed and typeset by David LeBlanc in Sabon 10.5/14
in Montreal, Quebec

CONTENTS

ABBREVIATIONS

APHA American Public Health Association
ACT Associated Canadian Travelers
AECL Atomic Energy Canada Limited
BCG Bacille Calmette Guérin vaccination (TB)
DOT Directly Observed Therapy
HSPC Health Services Planning Commission
IODE Imperial Order of the Daughters of the Empire
MBBCH Doctor of Medicine, Bachelor of Surgery
MRCP Member, Royal College of Physicians
NRC National Research Council
NWMP North West Mounted Police
RM Rural Municipality
RPN Registered Psychiatric Nurse
SAB Saskatchewan Archives Board
SARM Saskatchewan Association of Rural Municipalities
SCA Saskatchewan Cancer Agency

Abbreviations

SDCMH Saskatchewan Division, Canadian Mental Health Association
SHSP Saskatchewan Hospital Services Plan
SLA Saskatchewan Lung Association
UHD Union hospital district
VON Victorian Order of Nurses

ACKNOWLEDGMENTS

I am indebted to many people. Early in the process, Eleanor McKinnon, private secretary to Premier T.C. Douglas; Malcolm Taylor, former secretary to the Health Services Planning Commission; and Hon. Walter Smishek, former minister of health, provided interviews. Hon. Sylvia Fedoruk wrote the foreword and critiqued the chapter on high-voltage radiation. Joan Feather and Lester Jorgenson critiqued the chapter on the Swift Current Health Region, and provided additional information. Dr Colin Smith critiqued the chapter on psychiatry, and Drs Ian McDonald and Frank Coburn provided interviews. Pat Matthews gave me biographical material and a photograph of her late husband; Mrs. William Burak provided a small photo of her late husband. The Saskatchewan Archives Board provided most of the photographs. Michael West provided permission to use the copyrighted photograph of Malcolm Taylor. Time Inc. provided a reproduction of their 30 January 1939 cover.

Acknowledgments

Associated Medical Services Inc., through its Hannah Institute for the History of Medicine Program, kindly gave permission to use material from R.G. *Ferguson, Crusader Against Tuberculosis* (1941). *The Canadian Medical Association Journal* and the *Annals of the Royal College of Physicians and Surgeons* have each allowed use of portions of four of my copyrighted articles published in their journals, as cited individually in the references. Drs John W. Aldrich and Brian C. Lentle have allowed extensive use of the Houston and Fedoruk chapter in their 1995 book that marked the centennial of Röntgen's discovery of x-rays. The Canadian Broadcasting Corporation program *Ideas* kindly allowed use of three excerpts from the radio program of 5 December 1990. Zennon Slowski and Dr Donald S Houston solved my computer problems.

The entire manuscript was read critically by Allan E. Blakeney, Mary I. Houston, and J. Frank Roy, and by doctors Ronald M. Bremner, Louis Horlick, Stan Houston, and Robert Lampard. I am grateful for their insightful comments and corrections. Any residual errors or omissions are the responsibility of the author.

FOREWORD

Saskatchewan has been a leader in many aspects of health care. These developments arose from the co-operation and mutual help necessary among pioneer settlers, sparsely distributed in a relatively hostile environment. House-raising, barn-raising and the building of community amenities such as schools and curling rinks made it logical for other co-operative developments also to occur.

These accomplishments took place in an atmosphere of community, creativity, and trust. Individuals with foresight such as Drs Seymour, Ferguson, Blair and Johns helped Saskatchewan to lead the world. In *Steps on the Road to Medicare: Why Saskatchewan Led*, Stuart Houston reviews many of the exciting events in a story that reflects the strengths of Saskatchewan people.

Stuart, himself, is truly a part of Saskatchewan history. He served on the executive of the Canadian Society for the History of Medicine from 1979 to 1987, including two years as president. His published works in medicine and the history of medicine number 268, including three books, thirteen chapters in books (among these three chapters in *Pediatric Skeletal Radiology, 1991*), and sixty-five original scientific articles. His published works in ornithology and natural history number 532 including four books, thirty chapters in books, and 244 original papers. His interest in ornithology is legendary, especially in bird-banding – he and his wife, Mary, have banded over 120,000 birds of 205 species, with 3,100 recoveries.

Stuart is professor emeritus of medical imaging at the University of Saskatchewan. Our paths have intertwined over many years. We both took our schooling in the Yorkton area of Saskatchewan in the 1940s. For about twenty years, until my retirement in 1986, Stuart and I collaborated in teaching radiation physics, the "Stuart and Sylvia show," to first-year medical students at the University of Saskatchewan. When I was chancellor, it was my privilege to present him with a DLitt degree (1997), though he had taken no classes and written no exams. Most of the medical students appreciated him – he is the only medical doctor to be elected honourary president of the Student Medical Society three times, including in his last full year of teaching and practice.

Stuart received Saskatchewan's highest honour, the Saskatchewan Order of Merit, in 1992, and was made an Officer of the Order of Canada in 1993. In 1997, he was the fourth recipient of the Gold Medal from the Canadian Association of Radiologists. His most recent honourary degree was a DCnL, in 2002.

The Honourable Sylvia O. Fedoruk,
OC, SOM, DStJ, BA, MA, DSc, LLD, DHumL, FCCPM

Steps on the Road to Medicare

INTRODUCTION

"Medicare is considered to be the most valued social programme in Canada today. Canadians have rated it as their most important concern, ahead of programmes in employment and social welfare ... medicare is an essential part of Canada's national identity and part ... of what it means to be Canadian."[1]

Most of the steps that led to medicare were forged in Saskatchewan. The events described in this book changed the course of health care throughout Canada.

There is a certain danger in listing all the times Saskatchewan was "first," leaving me open to charges of hero-worship, bragging and jingoism. Yet I hope those connected with Saskatchewan will be proud of the recurring themes of co-operation, innovation, and rapid response to need throughout Saskatchewan's fifty-five-year history of health care.

But one question must somehow be addressed. Why was Saskatchewan so consistently the leader? Why not Alberta? Manitoba? Nova Scotia?

Allow me to begin with a vignette from my own experience. As an amateur medical historian who in most years meets with the men and women of the Canadian Society for the History of Medicine, I understand full well, from the experiences narrated by friends at these meetings, the need to question conventional wisdom, folk legends, and mythology.

I had been told many times that Tommy Douglas, premier of Saskatchewan, had okayed development of the world's first "cobalt bomb" to treat cancer after one visit from Allan Blair and Harold Johns. This story was surely partly legend, and perhaps apocryphal folklore? So, when I had the chance to hear the truth first-hand, I seized the opportunity.

T.C. Douglas was coming to Saskatoon to give a speech at a major New Democratic Party (NDP) banquet in February 1983. I phoned Peter Prebble, my NDP member of the legislative assembly, and asked whether I could be booked for a short interview with Douglas. Peter phoned back to say that his schedule was full, but that if my wife, Mary, and I would come to the banquet, we would be assigned to drive Douglas back to his lodgings at the Bessborough Hotel. We accepted this unusually innovative offer with alacrity.

I had met Douglas only a few times. The first time, when I was a student, he was a guest in my family home in Yorkton, together with his personal advisor and assistant Morris C. Shumiatcher. I have a vivid after-supper memory of these two men standing beside the fireplace, my six-foot-four father towering over both. Early in Douglas's career as Co-operative Commonwealth Federation (CCF) premier of

Saskatchewan, my father had been on the committee that negotiated payments to doctors for treating people receiving social assistance: the impoverished elderly, widows, and orphans. Later Dad served as one of three doctors nominated by the Saskatchewan College of Physicians and Surgeons on the Thompson Advisory Planning Committee on Medical Care. As a high-school student, I had typed some of his letters and briefs.

As I drove him back to the hotel, Douglas asked after my parents and spoke well of both, the rancor of the so-called "doctors' strike" in 1962 notwithstanding. Time was short and Douglas needed to go to bed. I asked my well-prepared questions, and as I remember it, the conversation went as follows:

CSH: Do you remember the day that Harold Johns and Allan Blair dropped into your office to ask for permission to use the "cobalt bomb" to treat cancer?

TCD: Yes, clearly, as if it were only yesterday.

CSH: Is it true they came unannounced, without an appointment?

TCD: Probably. I had an open-door policy, guided by my trusted secretary Eleanor McKinnon. [Later an interview with Miss McKinnon in Regina confirmed that unscheduled visits were the rule. Douglas made it a policy to help any Saskatchewan citizen. The system worked best without fixed appointments.][2]

CSH: Is it true that you listened to their "pitch," asked for an approximation of the probable cost, and that they then walked out of your office with a virtual carte blanche to proceed?

TCD: Yes.

CSH: Is it true that you made this decision without consulting your treasurer, Clarence Fines, or any member of your cabinet?

TCD: Absolutely.

CSH: Is it true that you made this important decision without consultation with any other medical doctors or physicists, or any outside agency?

TCD: I believe that to be true.

CSH: How did you justify making such a momentous decision on the spur of the moment?

TCD: Well, after all, I was both premier and minister of health.[3]

CSH: How did you have the courage to do this without consultation with anyone at all?

TCD: Well, it was easy. I had complete confidence in the knowledge and the integrity possessed by both men. They assured me that high voltage radiotherapy offered great promise in the treatment of cancer. Dr Allan Blair had come from Toronto to head up the leading cancer agency in North America. And Harold Johns! Why, when I attended Brandon College, Alfred Edward Johns was my mathematics teacher and my favourite professor. He had been a missionary in Chengtu [Chengdu], West China, until 1924. His son, Harold, had been born in China. I was both poor and undernourished. The osteomyelitis in my femur was chronic, would periodically break down and issue pus, and this ran me down. The Johns family took pity on me and often had me over for Sunday supper in a deliberate attempt to put some weight on my frame. It was evident that their son, Harold, showed unusual promise. So, with my close

personal knowledge of both men and my complete
faith in their integrity, my permission did not seem to
me to be a gamble at all.

I told the above story in March 2002 to Shirley Douglas on
a phone-in program on CBC radio, and she thanked me for
it. I don't think she really believed her father had been that
rash, making so important a decision so quickly. But the
story as told above is an example of a visionary in action.
Douglas was a leader, the "right man in the right place at
the right time," who moved events forward. He was one
part of the answer to "Why Saskatchewan led the way."

CHAPTER 1

SASKATCHEWAN HOSPITALS:
Off to a Slow Start

To maintain a little balance in an unabashed book of firsts, it seems only fair to admit that the area that became Saskatchewan in 1905 was slow off the mark – the advent of hospitals was delayed in comparison with adjacent Manitoba and Alberta.

Strangely, the first hospital established in what is now Saskatchewan was in one of the most inaccessible parts of the province, at Ile-à-la-Crosse. Three dedicated Sisters of Charity (Grey Nuns), Sisters Agnes, Boucher, and Pépin, arrived there in 1860 with Bishop Grandin after an arduous journey of fifty-seven days in an open barge from St Boniface. This was only fourteen years after Father Taché (later Bishop Taché) set up his mission among the natives and a few French-speaking trappers. The three sisters established a convent, a dispensary, and a mission school.[1] In 1873 they began the formal operation of a hospital.[2]

Later, with the construction of each North West Mounted Police barracks, a building was set aside as a hospital.

Fort Walsh in the Cypress Hills was first in 1875, followed by Qu'Appelle in 1881, Regina and Maple Creek in 1883, and Battleford and Prince Albert in 1884.[3] When Dr Augustus L. Jukes was appointed senior surgeon to the North West Mounted Police in 1880,[4] and stationed at Fort Walsh, he appointed a pharmacist as hospital steward.

In 1885, two temporary military hospitals were created to care for wounded men evacuated from the battles of the Riel Rebellion. The first was a frame building with forty beds erected at Moose Jaw by the government. The head nurse was Hannah Grier Coombs, known as Mother Hannah, who later founded the Anglican Sisterhood of St John the Divine. The second, Saskatoon's temporary base hospital with up to eighty patients, was staffed by Dr James Bell of Montreal, Miss Millar (head nurse of the Winnipeg General Hospital, on loan), Nurse Phoebe Parsons, and Nurse Elkin. When the last Saskatoon patients were evacuated to Winnipeg by river barge and steamer, via Grand Rapids, the southern half of present-day Saskatchewan was again without a hospital.[5]

The first public hospital, at Saltcoats, was too far ahead of its time. Built in 1896, it opened in 1897 with a resident medical superintendent, a matron, and three trained nurses (Figure 1–1). An early tragedy sullied its record on 4 January 1898. Nurse Biggins went to the basement carrying a coal oil lamp, which hit an overhead beam, broke, and set her clothes on fire. She died the next day. By year's end, only forty-nine in-patients had been treated, but 374 days of free treatment had been provided. With its record of bad luck, and so many patients unable to pay, the hospital was closed.[6]

When the railroad reached "Pile of Bones" in 1882, it became the capital city of the North-West Territories. Canada's governor general, the Marquis of Lorne, was asked to

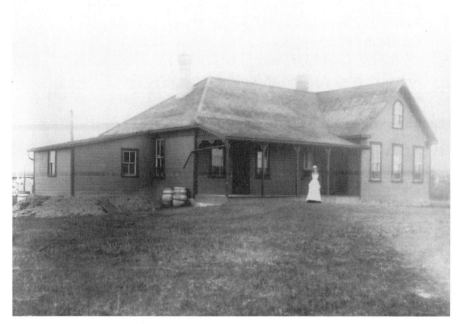

Figure 1–1 Saltcoats cottage hospital (SAB R-A23797)

give the new village a more suitable name. Since he was married to Queen Victoria's daughter, he christened it Regina in honour of his mother-in-law. Despite their town's designation as a capital city, Regina citizens requiring hospital care were forced to take the train east to Brandon or Winnipeg until late in 1889. That year the first general hospital in the North-West Territories opened in Medicine Hat with forty beds.[7] Regina patients alone accounted for 1,623 days of in-patient care in the Medicine Hat hospital in 1895.[8]

For nine years, Regina had only the Mary E. Truesdell Nursing Home, begun in August 1889. In 1896 the Regina branch of the National Council of Women began to raise money for a cottage hospital, with nurses supplied by the Victorian Order of Nurses (VON). The cottage hospital opened in 1898 (Figure 1–2).

Meanwhile, in Prince Albert, the Victoria Hospital began with a small building in 1899 (Figure 1–3). Its Ladies' Aid, among other contributions for the hospital, received night-shirts and a tablecloth, as well as a brace of Sharp-tailed Grouse, two dozen eggs, and six cakes to feed the patients.[9] At the conclusion of 1899 there were two hospitals, each with seven beds, to serve about 90,000 people.[10]

In 1899, the foundation was laid for a new twenty-five-bed hospital on Hamilton Street, just south of 14th Avenue in Regina. The VON contributed $1,500, with the proviso that the new hospital be named the Regina Victoria. Lady Minto, wife of the governor general, formally opened it in September 1901 (Figure 1–4). A nursing training school began at once, with three students in the first class. The hospital continued to expand and was taken over by the city of Regina in 1907. It has been the largest hospital in Saskatchewan ever since.

The third permanent hospital in southern Saskatchewan, the Queen Victoria Hospital (Figure 1–5), opened in my hometown of Yorkton in 1902, the drive for $1,800 sparked by one of my heroes, Dr T.A. Patrick. The VON contributed $3,000. Here began the second school of nursing. One of the graduates of this unaccredited school was Margaret Fraser. After her husband died, Margaret Fraser Myles took upgrading and returned to be matron of the Yorkton hospital in the late 1920s. She then moved to Aberdeen, Scotland, where she became the author of the world's best-selling *Textbook of Midwifery*, ten editions of which appeared between 1952 and 1985.[11]

The Moosomin hospital also opened in 1902 (Figure 1–6), the first hospital between Brandon and Regina.

The fifth and sixth hospitals opened in Maple Creek in 1904 and Indian Head (Figure 1–7) in 1905. Both had nursing training schools. Maple Creek began as an eight-bed cottage hospital, but moved into a twenty-bed brick building in 1908. Nursing training continued until 1925 at Indian Head and 1935 at Maple Creek.[12]

When Saskatchewan was proclaimed a province in 1905, there were six hospitals in operation, four of them with nursing schools. Their seventy-five beds served over 250,000 people. In the 1901 census, populations of the main towns were as follows: Regina 2,249, Prince Albert 1,785, Moose Jaw 1,558, Moosomin 868, Yorkton 700, Battleford 609, and Maple Creek 382. By 1906 two more centres had grown to more than 1,000 population: Saskatoon with 3,011 and Indian Head with 1,545 inhabitants. Two of the eleven new towns with between 500 and 918 people in 1906 (Battleford 824 and Swift Current 554) soon

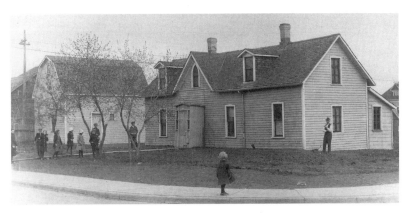

Figure 1–2 Victorian Order of Nurses Hospital, Regina (SAB R-B535)

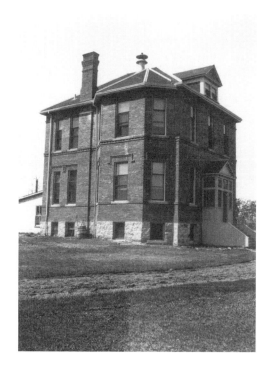

Figure 1–3
Victoria Hospital,
Prince Albert
(SAB R-A1679)

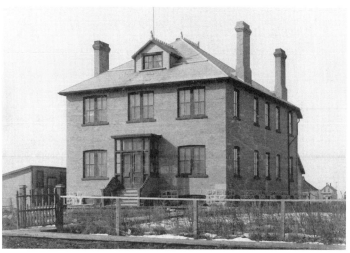

Figure 1–4 Regina Victoria Hospital, Regina (SAB R-B386)

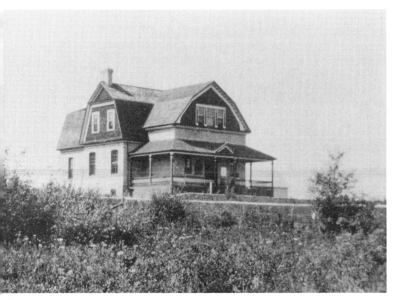

Figure 1–5 Queen Victoria Hospital, Yorkton
(Howard M. Jackson)

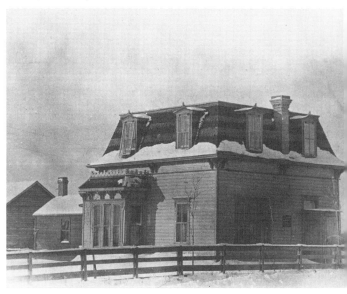

Figure 1–6 Moosomin Hospital (SAB R-A218)

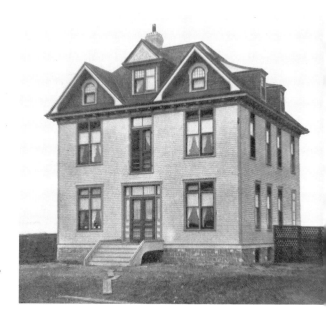

Figure 1–7
Lady Minto Hospital,
Indian Head
(SAB R-B10943)

built hospitals. Thus each centre with a population of 500 in 1900 or of 1,000 in 1906 had a hospital by 1912.

In 1906, a twenty-eight-bed, four-storey general hospital opened in Moose Jaw (Figure 1–8), just in time to care for victims of a typhoid epidemic. The building was steam-heated, but it had no elevator. That year a small rented building opened as a hospital in Lloydminster,[13] and the Presbyterian Church opened the Anna Turnbull Memorial Hospital (Figure 1–9) near their mission house in the hamlet of Wakaw.[14]

With the 1906 typhoid epidemic in the rapidly growing town of Saskatoon (which grew from 2,000 to 3,000 during the year), the eight beds in Nurse Sisley's nursing home (Figure 1–10) were quickly filled; cots were set up in surrounding buildings and even in the open grounds. The overflow of typhoid patients was taken to the new Roman Catholic rectory on Fifth Avenue, where Oblate Fathers Vachon and

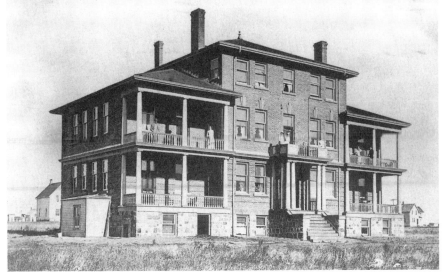

General Hospital. Moose Jaw. Sask.

Figure 1–8 General Hospital, Moose Jaw (SAB R-A7260)

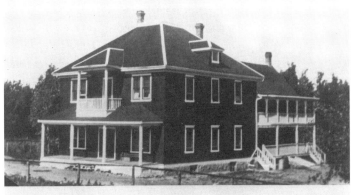

anna Turnbull Hospital, Wakaw Sask
1923

Figure 1–9 Anna Turnbull Memorial Hospital, Wakaw
(SAB R-A12696)

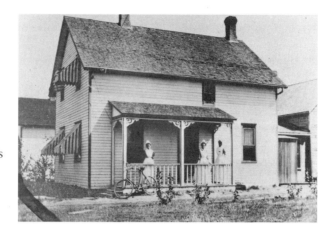

Figure 1–10
Nurse Sisley's
Nursing
Home,
Saskatoon
(A. Becker)

Paille cared for them around the clock. Propitiously, two Sisters of Charity from St Boniface came through Saskatoon in September. Although on a fundraising mission, they were pressed into service. In temporary quarters they cared for thirty-four severely ill typhoid patients, four of whom died. On 22 February 1907, the Grey Nuns purchased Dr J.H.C. Willoughby's private home on Pleasant Hill, just west of the Saskatoon city limits. They opened it with seventeen patient beds on 10 March 1907 (Figure 1–11).[15] A three-storey brick building was added in 1913 (Figure 1–12). A new Saskatoon City Hospital opened with fifty-six beds in April 1909; its official history claims it as the first municipal hospital in western Canada (Figure 1 13).[16]

In 1907 the Grey Nuns hospital was founded in Regina and the twenty-three-bed Lady Minto hospital, operated by the VON, opened in Melfort. The Womens' Missionary Society of the Presbyterian Church established a small hospital in Canora, which expanded to become the thirty-bed Hugh Waddell Memorial Hospital in 1914.

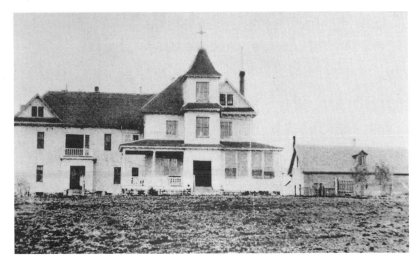

Figure 1–11 Dr J.H.C. Willoughby's home, Saskatoon
(A. Becker)

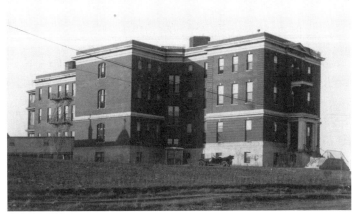

Figure 1–12 St Paul's Hospital, Saskatoon (SAB R-B1358)

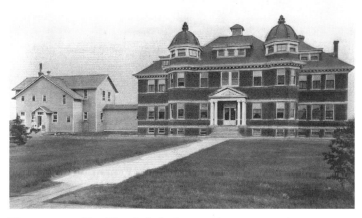

Figure 1–13 City Hospital, Saskatoon (SAB R-A3511)

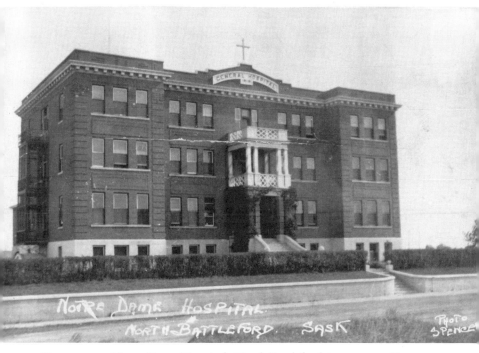

Figure 1–14 Notre Dame Hospital, North Battleford (SAB R-B5148)

The growing need for hospitals in other cities and towns was filled by Roman Catholic sisters. Sisters of Charity came from the Maritimes to open the twenty-five-bed Holy Family Hospital in Prince Albert in 1910, and Sisters of Providence came from Montreal to found Notre Dame Hospital in North Battleford in 1911 (Figure 1–14). In 1912, Sisters of St Elizabeth came from Austria to launch St Elizabeth's Hospital in Humboldt and Sisters of Providence of Kingston opened the thirty-bed Moose Jaw Providence Hospital in 1912.[17] That year, general hospitals opened in Swift Current (Fig. 1–15) and Weyburn (Fig. 1–16).[18] By 1912, in terms of hospital availability, Saskatchewan was beginning to catch up with its two neighbouring provinces.

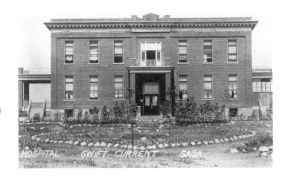

Figure 1–15
Swift Current
Hospital
(SAB R-A3351)

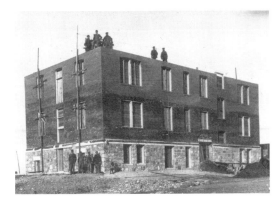

Figure 1–16
Municipal
Hospital,
Weyburn
(SAB R-B129)

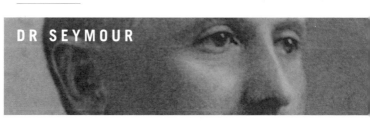

DR SEYMOUR

Maurice M. Seymour is the pacesetter in our story. Born 7 July 1857, in Goderich, Ontario, Seymour was one of three children of Captain Maurice Bain Seymour, who hailed from Ireland, and Maria MacDonald, who came from Scotland. He began his studies at Assumption College, Windsor, Ontario, in 1873 and then obtained his medical degree from McGill University in 1879. Rather unusually for those times, he took two years of post-graduate study before he went into practice.[1]

After employment with the Canadian Pacific Railway during its construction in 1881–83 and service in the Riel Rebellion in 1885, Seymour practised in the beautiful Qu'Appelle Valley, forty-five miles northeast of Regina. He moved to Regina one year before Saskatchewan's formal birth and spent the rest of his professional life in charge of public health in the new province. For his first seventeen years, public health had a low profile, as a mere branch within the large and powerful Department of Agriculture (under Hon. W.R. Motherwell), and then within Municipal Affairs. Whatever his title and whichever government department he worked within, Seymour laid a solid, achievement-filled, and logical foundation for public health. His enforcement arm was the Royal North West Mounted Police. In his new province in 1905, Seymour saw that financial aid, 50 cents per patient day, was needed for the six hospitals – in Prince Albert (1899), Regina (1901), Yorkton and Moosomin (1902), and Battleford and Indian Head (1905).

One of Seymour's strengths was his ability to react rapidly to provincial needs by drafting forward-looking legislation that would receive support from members of both political parties. Some of his actions were firsts for Canada. Responding quickly to the needs of the Rural Municipality (RM) of Sarnia #221, which had used $1,500 of tax money in 1915 to retain Dr Schmitt in that community (see chapter 3), the legislature the very next year amended the Municipalities Act to allow use of municipal taxes to build a hospital, hire a nurse, or expend up to $1,500 to hire a doctor – a first in North America.

Seymour also drafted Saskatchewan's Venereal Disease Act in 1920, with a revision in 1923. This was not a first in Canada, for Alberta had passed its own act and had begun offering free treatment in 1918. Venereal disease (VD, now known as Sexually Transmitted Infection) was relatively common, particularly syphilis. Saskatchewan offered free diagnosis and treatment. On a single day in 1924, in Regina, the VD clinic treated 100 adults, half of them for syphilis and half for gonorrhea, and five children for congenital syphilis.[2]

In 1912, only one birth in twenty occurred in hospital. By 1923 this figure had risen to one in six. The "Maternity Grant" of $25 in 1914 was designed by Seymour as a boon to farm women in particular, providing $15 for the attending physician and $10 for clothes and bedclothes for the baby.[3] In 1920, seventeen mothers applied; in 1921, 125; in 1922, 253; in 1923, 286; and in 1924, 427.[4]

By 1923, there were 2,253 hospital beds in a province of 770,000, or nearly three beds per thousand population. Since people were often quite sick before they entered hospital, it is not surprising that the average stay was 12.7 days.[5]

One of the biggest public health problems was tuberculosis (TB). Soon after Seymour's son was treated at the famous Trudeau Sanatorium at Saranac Lake, New York, Seymour organized the public meeting on 17 February 1911 that formed the Saskatchewan Anti-tuberculosis League. He persuaded the League to build its first sanatorium in an attractive coulee nestled in the Qu'Appelle Valley, facing Echo Lake and protected from north winds. At that time, bovine tuberculosis caused 25% of TB deaths among Saskatchewan children; 18% of 456,000 cattle tested were positive for TB.[6] Eventually, Seymour achieved uniform, free tuberculin testing of cattle.

On the advice of Dr D.A. Stewart of Ninette, Manitoba, Seymour hired Dr R.G. Ferguson to run the province's tuberculosis program.

With typhoid fever, bovine tuberculosis, and summer dysentery all taking a toll, the Canadian Public Health Association appointed Seymour chairman of a country-wide study of milk problems in Canada from 1924 through 1926. Seymour's group sent fifty-two questions to every Canadian city with a population over 20,000 and published the results.[7]

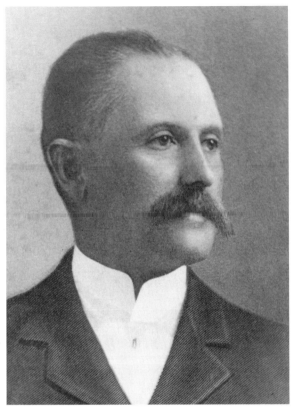

Figure 2–1 Dr Maurice M. Seymour (SLA)

They reported that Canada's per capita milk consumption was 0.4 litres/day (compared to New York City at 0.3). More deaths in Canada were due to milk than to any other food. For example, there were 42 deaths from 619 instances of typhoid and scarlet fever and an unknown number due to tuberculosis, all presumed to have been transmitted by milk. Dr E.W. Stapleford, president of Regina College, told a hearing about the deaths of 8 of his 204 students and 1 of his teachers from raw milk delivered daily from a farm a few miles outside Regina. Stapleford described "nine coffins being carried out."[8]

Saskatchewan led in the tuberculin testing of cattle. In April 1917, the City of Saskatoon was the first in Canada to inspect and license all dairy herds supplying the city; cows were tested by the Dominion Health of Animals Branch. Five other Saskatchewan cities and four towns followed. An additional thirty-one towns and seventy villages had organized preliminary inspection and licensing. Seymour recommended pasteurization of milk (heating to $142-145°F$ for thirty minutes, then cooling until delivered), but his suggestion was difficult to implement during hot summer days.

Diphtheria was another serious problem; in 1917, Seymour began giving out free antitoxin to be dispensed by the medical profession.

Seymour was not an unduly modest man (Figure 2–1). In 1926 he published his Atlantic City presidential address to the Conference of State and Provincial Health Authorities under the title "The Seymour Plan." He asked general practitioners to immunize against diphtheria in September and October, smallpox during November and December, and typhoid during January and February.[9] He tried to make public health simple and easy to understand, with such slogans as "Do not spit" and "Swat the fly."

Cancer increased steadily during his tenure, until it edged out tuberculosis by exactly one death in 1924. That year, however, Saskatchewan had the lowest general death rate of any portion of the British Empire.[10]

Seymour was a member of the North-West Territories Medical Council from 1885 to 1905 and served twice as president. He organized the Saskatchewan Medical Association in 1906. He was one of the first in Canada to obtain a diploma in public health from the University of Toronto. In 1915 he served as president of the Canadian Public Health Association and as vice-president of the American Public Health Association (APHA). In 1923 he represented Canada at the Health Section, League of Nations. In 1925 he was elected president of the Conference of State and Provincial Health Authorities. He was honoured as a fellow of the Royal Institute of Public Health in England, a fellow of APHA, and a recipient of an honourary LLD degree from the University of Ottawa in 1925. Dr Lillian Chase described him as "a great organizer, a man of varied gifts and charming personality, [who] enjoyed the esteem of all."[11]

Why was Seymour so successful in a province with limited resources in such difficult times? He was a capable administrator, with unceasing energy. His greatest strength was his ability to harness Saskatchewan's highly developed co-operative spirit. He could achieve support from municipal councils (in enforcing health laws for the common good, even when this might seem elsewhere to impinge too much on personal freedom); teachers (one year he sent a letter to each teacher in the province); clergymen (when launching a vaccination campaign, he would ask that an announcement be read from the pulpit on the preceding Sunday); rural Homemakers' Clubs (who assisted gratis the doctors and nurses during his vaccination campaigns), and weekly newspapers (which published his weekly article on health).

Seymour was not superannuated until 1 November 1927, at age seventy, when he became medical advisor to the government on public health matters. His greatest gift to the people of Saskatchewan was his unbelievably rapid response to the grassroots development of municipal doctors and municipal hospitals. He also laid a sound foundation for Saskatchewan's future leadership in health.

He died on 16 January 1929, at seventy-one, fifteen days after Saskatchewan initiated the first universal free treatment for tuberculosis, the next stepping stone on the road to medicare.

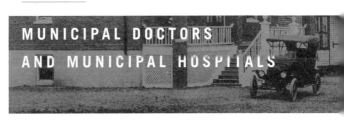

CHAPTER 3

MUNICIPAL DOCTORS
AND MUNICIPAL HOSPITALS

The first municipal doctor in North America:
Dr Henry Schmitt of Holdfast, 1915
One major step on the road to medicare occurred in the RM
of Sarnia. The Holdfast history book, *History and Heritage,*
quotes the motion passed by the council of the Rural
Municipality of Sarnia #221 in January 1914: "That Council advertise for a doctor ... Also first correspond with Dr
Schmitt of Newton, Illinois, in regard to locating here."
Perhaps Schmitt wrote to Holdfast in response to adver-
tisements which talked of "The Last Great West" and the
"Beautiful Last Mountain Valley where crop failures are
unknown,"[1] or the contact may have been made by a
farmer who had moved from Illinois, lured by the promise
of free land in Saskatchewan. In the Sarnia Council minutes
of 25 June 1914 it is recorded that Dr Schmitt of Holdfast
was "appointed Medical Health Officer for the village to
take effect on 1 July and that Dr Chapman of Dilke [should]
be notified to that effect."[2]

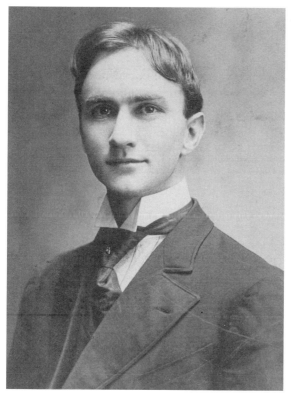

Figure 3–1 Dr H.J. Schmitt, graduation photo
(Mary Bradshaw)

According to the Holdfast history, "Dr Schmitt covered great distances to minister to the sick" (Figure 3–1). Since the RM of Sarnia included nine townships and most roads were prairie trails, his early mode of travel was horse and gig in summer, and horse and cutter in winter. In 1915, he bought a model T Ford for summer travel when roads permitted.[3] That year Dr Schmitt had difficulty collecting enough money from the impoverished farmers and considered moving on to the larger and more prosperous community of Craik.[4] Because the people of the municipality were much concerned, the Sarnia council agreed to vote funds from tax money to pay a retainer to Dr Schmitt. This agreement was the first municipal doctor arrangement in North America.[5] To keep Schmitt in the community, the rural municipality paid him a stipend of $1,500 in 1915 and $2,500 in 1916.[6] The Honourable George Langley, minister of agriculture in charge of health matters, wrote to RM Sarnia, "We watch your experiment hopefully but skeptically." But as the Holdfast history recorded, Langley "need not have worried. Every settler in the area would soon attest to the fact that Dr Schmitt's services far outweighed the remuneration he received."[7]

First municipal doctor legislation in North America, 1916
In 1916 the Saskatchewan Legislature, influenced by Seymour, enacted the Municipal Hospital Act, permitting rural municipalities to make a grant to physicians to supplement income, such grant not to exceed $1,500. This made legal what RM Sarnia had already done. In 1919, legislation was enacted whereby a rural municipality might engage a physician on a salary – not to exceed $5,000 – to provide free medical care to the residents of the municipality. In 1932, provision was made whereby portions of municipalities might engage the services of a physician, or two or more municipalities could co-operate. By 1935, provision was made in the Town and Village acts for an assessment of up to $2 per head of population, according to the last Dominion census, to engage a physician. In 1937, a further change permitted the raising of a sum of $5,000 for a surgeon. Finally, in 1941, the Rural Municipality Act was amended to permit physicians to be paid on a fee-for-service basis from public funds.

How successful were the municipal doctor plans?
A helpful source of information is the report of the Committee on Municipal Physicians, presented by Dr D.S. Johnstone, a Regina surgeon, to the Canadian Medical Association annual meeting in Regina in 1927. That year there were thirteen municipal doctors in Saskatchewan, practising in twelve localities: Holdfast, Craik, Beechy,[8] Bethune, Birsay, Brock, Chamberlain, Freemont, Leroy, Lintlaw, Rush Lake, and Senlac. Most municipal doctors were paid between $3,500 and $5,000. All medical needs of ratepayers and their hired help were covered. The Johnstone committee stated that Craik and Holdfast were "old and well settled municipalities, where the practice was quite able to sustain one or more doctors in each municipality – it was apparently a straight case of going out to hire a doctor in the hope of saving money [and] attendance fees."[9]

The municipal doctor system attracted the interest of the Committee on the Costs of Medical Care in the United States. They sent C. Rufus Rorem, an economist, to study the situation in 1929 and 1930. His studies resulted in an eighty-four-page book in 1931.[10] Rorem's map (Figure 3–2) showed the location of the thirty-two municipalities with municipal doctors in Saskatchewan.[11] Twenty employed twenty-one full-time doctors; twelve other municipalities had part-time agreements with sixteen physicians.[12] Seven municipalities engaged municipal doctors for the first time in 1929 while another four did so in 1930. In 1930, Saskatchewan had 558 licensed practitioners and a total hospital bed capacity of 3,357, but only one of the municipal doctors had a hospital to work in. Of Saskatchewan

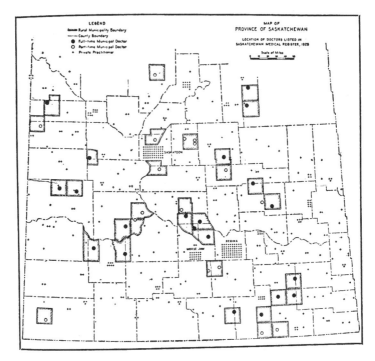

Figure 3-2 Rorem's map of where municipal doctors were located in Saskatchewan (courtesy University of Chicago Press)

inhabitants, 69% lived on farms, 9% in 377 villages, 7% in 80 towns, and 15% in eight cities with a population of 5,000 people or more.[13]

Rorem found that most doctors were pleased with the system because their incomes were assured. Annual salaries ranged from $2,800 to $5,000, but the doctors were responsible for paying automobile and office upkeep. The statistics collected by Rorem, who did not name any of his informants, showed that one doctor made 426 country calls in a year, necessitating travel of 5,580 miles by automobile.

Most municipal doctors pocketed an initial charge of $1 to $3 for the first call; they were allowed to charge mileage for such visits and an extra $7 for obstetrical care. One municipality allowed a doctor to charge $7 for simple fractures, and another allowed a fixed fee of $5 for minor operations.

One insurmountable difficulty facing municipal doctors was the complete rigidity of the Federal Income Tax Division, which insisted on treating the entire income as salary. Even though each doctor had to maintain an office, equipment, and an automobile, these costs could not be deducted as expenses because the Income Tax Division viewed municipal doctors as salaried employees. The medical profession was unable to obtain any redress of this unfair practice, except for a few municipalities which reimbursed expenses separately from the stipend.[14]

Despite this, most doctors who had previously been in private practice reported that bad debts had so reduced their cash incomes that they were better off with the annual salary of the municipal scheme, although they worked harder after the impediment of the patient's financial status was removed. One doctor told Rorem, "I am lucky to be on a salary." Several stated that freedom from financial worries improved the quality of their service to patients and that patients co-operated by seeking services earlier in an illness. On the other hand, some doctors felt insecure because they could be dismissed on three months' notice. Several felt that state medicine would not be appropriate outside the special rural situation. One doctor mentioned three families who tended to abuse the scheme, but admitted that they would have been a nuisance to a doctor under any payment system. Physicians agreed that the plan did not interfere with the doctor-patient relationship, and that they could spend more time on prevention, such as vaccination programs. Each municipal doctor served as medical health officer for the municipality and the villages within it. One reported that this was the first year in which there were no cases of diphtheria in his municipality, a situation he attributed to his intensive vaccination program.

Municipal officials were even more enthusiastic; one of them said, "If you get a good man who is interested in his work and the health of the municipality, the system cannot be beat." Another said, "The municipal physician's system is here to stay, for the simple reason that it works out to the benefit of both parties concerned." One official reported that this was the first time he had seen *all* taxpayers satisfied over a rise in taxes.[15] In one municipality the candidate for reeve (the rural equivalent of mayor), who ran for office in 1928 on a platform of discontinuing the municipal doctor plan, was defeated by 231 to 30 votes. In another municipality, at the annual ratepayers' meeting, a taxpayer moved that the council dismiss the present municipal doctor, but no one seconded his motion.[16] No individual patient was heavily burdened, yet the taxation basis recognized the difference in financial ability to pay, since the more land one held, the more one paid. Only a few large landowners complained.[17] Once the municipal doctor system had been adopted, no community returned to a private practice basis. The only downside was that the presence of municipal physicians had unfavourable economic effects upon the practice of independent physicians in adjoining towns and cities.[18]

Municipal doctors worked hard. Dr Schmitt's successor at Holdfast in the early 1930s was Dr C.S. McLean. Each year in the early 1930s McLean drove 14,000 miles to make

1,400 house calls, saw another 1,500 patients in his office, and attended fifty to seventy maternity cases.[19]

A circular sent by the United Farmers of Canada, Local Council, to taxpayers of one municipality before a vote on introducing the municipal doctor system there stated:

At present we are committing to pooling our wheat and other farm products. The municipal doctor scheme is in reality a pooling of our doctors bills ... an insurance against unduly high doctor bills in any one year – an equalization scheme. Are you willing to invest $4.50 per quarter section in the health of our section of the nation? A nation's first wealth is health, and levies to protect our first wealth should have priority over all others.[20]

Things got worse for those doctors not under a municipal plan. The minister of health reported that the "average cash earnings of 130 doctors in the drought area, over a period of two years," was $27 a month.[21] In order to retain these doctors in the province, the Saskatchewan government provided a monthly relief payment of $75 to those in the most drought-stricken areas, a program that continued for five years.[22]

To oversee and regulate the municipal doctor system, the Health Services Board was set up, with equal representation from the province, the Saskatchewan Association of Rural Municipalities (SARM), and the College of Physicians and Surgeons.[23]

By October 1938, at the time of Dr R.G. Ferguson's report on municipal doctor schemes to the Saskatchewan Medical Association, 121 of the 546 provincial doctors were under remarkably varied types of municipal contract. For example, 28 received the $1,500 retainer grant, 36 received a salary of up to $5,000 for regular medical services, and 13 had a contract to supply surgery within the competence of the doctor. In only 15 instances was a physician permitted to charge a flat $2 deterrent fee for the first call, and a reduced fee for maternity cases, fractures, and surgery. Of 546 private family practitioners in the province, 121 cared for ninety-two municipalities, two towns and forty-two villages, a total of 116,421 persons in a Saskatchewan population of 930,893 (12.5%).[24] In 1937, the average amount owing the doctor by the municipality was $2,503, while one drought-stricken municipality owed its doctor $13,387.60 in unpaid salary.[25]

In 1941 Dr John J. Collins, a municipal doctor at Ituna, sent a questionnaire to Saskatchewan rural doctors; ninety replied. They were almost unanimous in declaring that private practice was no longer feasible. One replied, "Any system is to be preferred to the present. Collections appear hopeless. I do not know how medical men can hope to carry on out here [all year] under present and future conditions." In 1941, municipal doctors reported a mean net income of $3,290, after expenses of $2,012, for serving, on average, 1,998 people (roughly $2 per capita). Thirty percent of income was privately earned, mainly from treating patients from outside the municipality.[26]

By 1942, a model contract was drawn up by the Health Services Board of the Saskatchewan College of Physicians and Surgeons. Each municipal doctor was to be paid at the rate of one cent per day per quarter section, $432 per township, or $3,888 for a nine-township municipality. This payment was to be for 300 days in any calendar year, the doctor to have all Sundays and statutory holidays off. This was a striking departure from tradition, whereby rural doctors were on call twenty-four hours a day, seven days a week. For country calls, the model contract suggested that doctors be paid ten cents per mile each way by car in summer, fifteen cents from 1 November to 31 March, twenty cents for snowmobile travel and thirty cents per mile each way for a horse-drawn vehicle.[27]

In 1944, there were at least 101 municipal doctors in Saskatchewan. By the peak year of 1947, they cared for 210,000 people, nearly a quarter of the population.[28] In 1950, there were still 173 municipal doctors in Saskatchewan.[29] Since the municipal doctor system offered immediate guaranteed payment, it was often preferred by young doctors in their first few years of practice. They saw it as an alternative to "starving" in a city while they built up a practice against competition, and waited months or years for patients to pay their bills.

The municipal doctor system was beneficial for patients as well, since it encouraged doctors to practice in rural areas. When medicare was introduced in Saskatchewan on 1 July 1962, the need for salaried municipal doctor schemes vanished. With immediate payment from the provincial government, new doctors could begin practice in a city; as a result, totally unplanned and unforeseen by government, many a village, especially one without a hospital, soon lost its doctor. The trend for doctors to cluster in the cities accelerated.

Municipal doctor schemes were developed locally in response to need. The councillors of the rural municipality of Sarnia deserve much credit for an innovative idea quickly put into practice; Seymour merits recognition for his rapid response in making it legal. Municipal doctors were another step on the road to medicare.

First legislation in North America to allow Union Hospital Districts

Municipal hospital programs paralleled those for municipal doctors, but require separate mention. In 1916, legislative provision was made "for the combining of towns, villages and rural municipalities in union hospital districts" (UHDs) to erect and maintain a hospital. By 1920, there were ten UHDs in Saskatchewan;[30] by 1930, twenty; by the early 1940s, twenty-six.[31]

Alberta was not far behind in this respect, with its first municipal hospital in the village of Mannville in 1919, followed quickly by hospitals in Bassano, Cardston, Drumheller, Islay, Onoway, Vermilion, and Lloydminster, the last shared with Saskatchewan.[32] By 1922, hospitals were added in Hanna, High River and Provost. Capital, maintenance, and operation were provided by the people in the district: the only revenue received from the Alberta government was a grant of fifty cents per day per patient.[33]

In Saskatchewan, the Sigerist report in 1944 (chapter 5) gave sudden impetus to building new hospitals and to forming new Union Hospital Districts[34] – forty-four new UHDs were created in three years. By 1947, the seventy-eight UHDs "covered more than one-third of the settled area of the province, included approximately one-third of the population, and provided about three-eighths of the ... hospital beds."[35]

First municipal hospital legislation in Canada

As an exception to the long lists of other "firsts," municipal hospital legislation priority was shared between Alberta and Saskatchewan in the border city of Lloydminster. Here the local hospital, opened in 1906, closed for financial reasons in 1912. David Grieve Tuckwell, editor of the *Lloydminster*

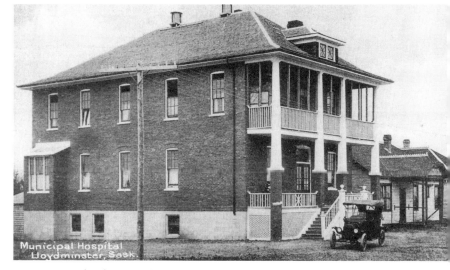

Figure 3–3 Lloydminster Union Hospital (SAB S-B150)

Times and a new arrival from Australia, promoted the idea of a union hospital, supported by the town and six surrounding municipalities. The hospital reopened in October 1913 (Figure 3–3). Rural municipality residents contributed one cent per acre; Tuckwell proudly noted that the homesteader, and his wife, family, and dependents, gained hospital accommodation for $1.60 per year, the "very maximum of protection for the very minimum of cost."[36]

In 1916, Alberta and Saskatchewan each passed appropriate legislation. In the latter province it read: "The Council of the Town of Lloydminster, the Rural Municipality of Britannia and the Rural Municipality of Wilton may enter into agreement with each other to provide money for the maintenance and extension of the said hospital and for the payment of the [hospital] expenses of their respective ratepayers and residents."[37] The legislation served as an example for other areas.

Saskatchewan passed a more general Union Hospital Act in 1917. To improve and streamline administration, the Rural Municipality Act was amended in 1927, 1928, 1929, and 1934. The Village Act and the Town Act were amended in 1936.[38] In 1939, an "umbrella act," the Municipal Medical and Hospital Services Act, was passed.[39]

By 1948, eighty-eight municipalities provided their residents with hospital service at municipal expense. Sixty-six financed this through a property tax and twelve utilized the Municipal Medical and Hospital Services Act, which allowed a personal tax.[40] By 1954, there were 104 union hospital districts.[41]

First legislation in Canada to allow personal taxation for health purposes
Previously, health services could be financed only by a tax on property. In 1934, the Rural Municipality Act[42] "was amended to empower the council to fix an annual tax for non-ratepayers. This appears to be the first instance in which statutory authority was granted for the levying of a personal tax for health services ... in Canada." As Taylor says, "the construction and maintenance of hospital facilities and the prepayment of medical and hospital services through municipal tax levies – are a tribute to local initiative and the understanding of the importance of health services ... a remarkable development not duplicated on such a scale elsewhere in Canada."[43] Once again, Saskatchewan residents worked together to give health a top priority, to a degree not seen in the rest of the country.

CHAPTER 4

DR FERGUSON AND TUBERCULOSIS

In fighting the disease that for many years took the greatest toll on health and productivity, Robert George Ferguson was one of the most consistent and effective leaders in North America. Sixth in a family of sixteen, he was born on 12 September 1883 near the Red River at Joliette, North Dakota, only seventeen miles south of the forty-ninth parallel. At age nineteen he was delegated by his family to choose a farm in Saskatchewan, of similar size to the one being vacated in North Dakota. He selected one at the south edge of Yorkton and moved his parents, brothers, and sisters there. Four years later his father died. George managed the farm in summer and attended Wesley College in Winnipeg in winter, obtaining his BA in 1910, intending a career in the ministry. When his husky voice, due to childhood diphtheria, did not allow him to preach three sermons each Sunday, he chose medicine as next best, graduating with his MD in 1916 (Figure 4–1).[1]

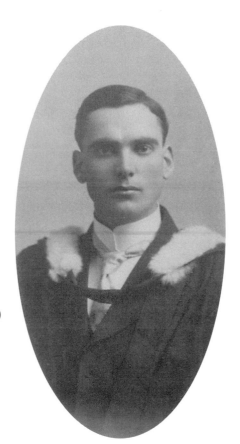

Figure 4–1
Dr R.G. Ferguson,
graduation photo (SLA)

Ferguson's interest in research stemmed from his student experience in Dr S.J.S. Pierce's laboratory in Winnipeg, making typhoid vaccine for Canadian troops in World War I. His interest in tuberculosis had been stimulated by his work, while still a medical student, with Dr D.A. Stewart, medical superintendent at the Ninette Sanatorium in Manitoba. Stewart had so much faith in Ferguson's integrity and ability that he left him, still a final year medical student, in administrative charge of the sanatorium for a few weeks to go on his honeymoon.

Ferguson's first year in medical practice in Winnipeg under Dr A.B. Alexander was the best possible preparation for his later career, with first-hand responsibility at the King George, the infectious disease hospital, and the King Edward, the city's tuberculosis hospital. During 1916–17 he developed his three postulates of tuberculosis control:

1 Early discovery means early recovery.
2 Reduce the level of infection in the community.
3 Interrupt the transmission of the tubercle bacillus.

As Dr G.D. Barnett later commented, these three postulates became the foundation on which the Saskatchewan program was built.

In July 1917, Ferguson was appointed acting superintendent of the new sanatorium at Fort Qu'Appelle, Saskatchewan (Figure 4–2), on the recommendation of Dr Stewart. Almost immediately the site became known as Fort San; a full post office by that name existed in the administration building from 1926 to 1966. As the only doctor, Ferguson was on call twenty-four hours a day; he was known to sit up all night holding the hand of a dying patient. In 1919, he attracted two equally dedicated assistants, Dr Harvey Boughton and Dr R.W. Kirkby, whom Ferguson later promoted to direct the new sanatoria in Saskatoon (15 April 1925) and Prince Albert (7 January 1930), respectively.

At that time, tuberculosis was epidemic among the Indian population. It was also much the commonest cause of death in white adults between the ages of twenty and forty-five,[2] killing or disabling more able-bodied wage earners and homemakers than did heart disease, cancer, or other infections. Before the widespread advent of x-ray machines,

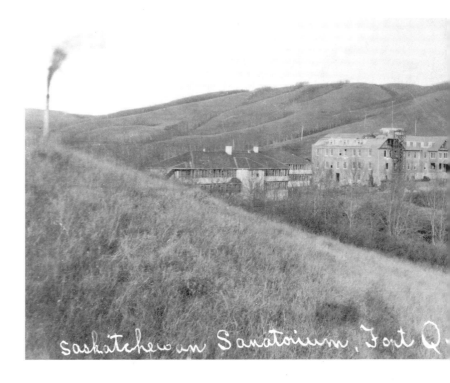

Saskatchewan Sanatorium, Fort Q.

symptoms were insidious and non-specific; many patients were in the advanced stage before a correct diagnosis was made. Poverty, overcrowding of large families in small prairie shacks, and malnutrition favoured tuberculosis and in turn led to more poverty. The disease spread through coughing and by the unregulated sale of milk from infected cows.

First in grassroots public support, 1917–48
Nowhere else in North America did the attack on tuberculosis, or perhaps any other single disease, have as much

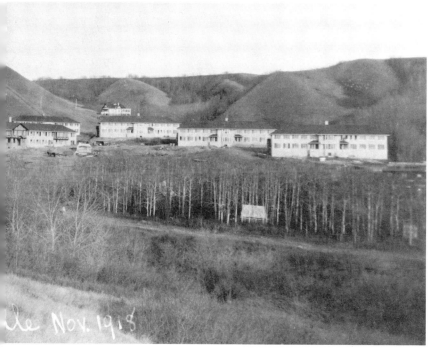

Figure 4-2 Fort Qu'Appelle Sanatorium (SLA)

grassroots support. In spite of the apparently unpromising outlook, Ferguson galvanized, educated, and cajoled an entire province.

He harnessed the co-operative spirit needed for survival in a new province with poor roads and harsh winters. Rural communities were fertile ground for his persuasive talents. Under his guidance, schoolchildren, teachers, nurses, doctors, service clubs, municipalities, and the provincial government co-operated in a costly but seemingly effective effort, unequalled anywhere else on the continent. The aims were to raise money for the Anti-tuberculosis League and to keep public concern alive. Often the responses were simple, but symbolic. Groups of farmers' wives, scattered throughout the province and organized as Homemakers' Clubs, would each donate dozens of eggs or chickens to feed patients. The Imperial Order of the Daughters of the Empire, better known as the IODE, made tuberculosis its main concern; members raised money to build the children's pavilion, furnish the schoolroom, buy books for the library, pay the bills of indigent children, and build and staff a preventorium, where mothers could be isolated from their infants from birth.[3] Radio announcers donated their time to put on weekly amateur shows. There was an annual tuberculosis essay contest for schoolchildren. Prospective teachers were taught about tuberculosis at Normal School, the name then given to the Teachers' College.

Twice, snowstorms led to important, long-term fundraising activities. Ferguson's timing in each instance was impeccable. In 1934, his car was stuck in the snow and he walked to a railroad car on the track nearby. In it were members of the newly formed Associated Canadian Travelers (ACT), a group searching for a public service project. When they heard Ferguson's needs, they agreed to help in the annual Christmas Seal campaign. On another occasion, other ACT members, stormbound with Ferguson in Nipawin, agreed to try amateur radio broadcasts as a means of raising money, and eventually broadcast these over six stations for more than thirty years. The ACT raised $813,000 to combat TB between 1934 and 1955.[4]

In a predominantly rural province, Ferguson, as a son of the farm, understood farmers and spoke their language. He represented the anti-tuberculosis campaign by an agrarian metaphor in his 1942 annual report:

The people of Saskatchewan know that tuberculosis is a bad weed. In the language of the farmer, it is a perennial which, if not uprooted, will shed its seeds from year to year. When these weeds or cases are sparse the best practice is to find them and remove them before the seeds are shed. To do this everyone must learn to identify tuberculosis in the seed, in the sprout, in the leaf, in the flower, or in the ripe shelling. That is why the educational campaign for the prevention of tuberculosis goes on in schools, Normal Schools, families, communities, and throughout the province generally. From past results our people have the faith, confidence and will to eradicate this disease. Come peace, come war, prosperity or depression, this life-saving campaign goes on, resulting in less infection, less new cases, and in the end less deaths.[5]

In the early years Ferguson made certain that both legislators and doctors were familiar with the sanatorium and its work. On 26 November 1920, he gave a tour of the sanatorium to thirty members of the legislative assembly, and in June 1922 the Saskatchewan Medical Association held its annual meeting at the Fort Qu'Appelle Sanatorium.

After I published Ferguson's biography, I learned of another method he used to ensure legislative awareness. As superintendent, based at Fort Qu'Appelle, he was required to pay a monthly visit to the other two sanatoria, in Saskatoon and Prince Albert. Depending on whether he felt the premier (J.G. Gardiner, 1926–29 and 1934–35) or the minister of health (Dr J.M. Uhrich of Rosthern, 1923–29 and 1934–44) most required some gentle prodding, Ferguson would have his secretary telephone that person's secretary in Regina to learn when the dignitary was travelling north and on which train (there were four a day to Saskatoon). Ferguson would then be sure he was in Regina in time to catch the same train. This would give him three hours (four-and-a-half hours in the case of Health Minister Uhrich, if he was destined for his home constituency at Rosthern) to chat. Thus those in authority, the decision-makers, knew all about the problems and needs of all three sanatoria, the monthly field clinics in each major city and town, and so on. No person in a position such as Ferguson's in our faster, busier age has the slightest hope for such close personal contact with those in authority.

Ferguson was a rare person, superb in every aspect of his work. He had skills in teaching, clinical work, and research, and was also talented in administration and public relations. He knew exactly how to comfort the suffering, homesick, and lonesome. In his quiet way, by example and conviction, he taught everyone who came in contact with him and his work: doctors, nurses, medical students, patients and their families, and the general public.

Ferguson was one of the first sanatorium administrators in Canada to give a high priority to continuing education for his medical staff. Even when the San was hopelessly in debt during years of drought and depression, even when short-handed during wartime, he sent his staff away to learn. In spite of the time and expense to get there, London, England, was one of the most popular destinations because of its renowned teachers and the wealth of clinical experience available. Members of the medical staff often took an entire year of post-graduate training at the sanatorium's expense; each year at least one sanatorium physician went away for special studies. Training was sometimes rewarded by success in the Royal College of Physicians (MRCP) examination.[6]

Over the years, this education proved to be a good investment. Radiographers, nurses, and dietitians were regularly sent away for short courses and practical experience in another institution. There was no requirement of years of service to become eligible for further education. If the sanatorium needed someone trained in a new technique and a young staff member was eager to learn, an educational opportunity was available after only one or two years of employment.

Dr Harvey Boughton was the first to take educational leave; he spent two weeks in Winnipeg in 1920. Next, Ferguson went to Boston for two months in 1920; he spent one month studying heart disease with Dr Paul White, a world-renowned cardiologist, and three weeks taking a $100 course in internal medicine at Harvard University. Ferguson believed that the physician who is limited to treating one disease is "apt to develop a blind side, and to lose his true perspective in the interpretation of symptoms which are the common stock of widely different diseases."[7] To recognize early tuberculosis, one had to keep in touch with the whole field of internal medicine. In Boston, one of the first centres to provide courses for graduates in medicine, alongside a splendid medical library, a doctor's medical experience and perspectives could be broadened.

Later, Ferguson arranged for every student nurse in Saskatchewan to attend an eight-week affiliation course at a sanatorium. Between 1 June 1945 and May 1964, 3,774 student nurses had this practical experience at either the Fort Qu'Appelle or the Saskatoon sanatorium. Transportation and sickness expenses were paid by the sanatoria. The affiliate nursing course ended at Fort San in October 1962 and at the Saskatoon San in May 1964.

Writing his own ticket: The Saskatchewan Anti-tuberculosis Commission (1921–22)

Ferguson was an unassuming, soft-spoken, compassionate doctor. His personal charm, vision, strength of purpose, and scientific methodology were to make him a leader in North America's fight against tuberculosis.

His quiet influence with the premier and the Department of Health and his compelling persuasiveness worked wonders. He had a lifelong knack for getting what he wanted from governments.

After only four years as head of the tuberculosis program, Ferguson convinced the powers-that-be that little was known about the disease anywhere in North America. He persuaded the government to form the Saskatchewan Anti-tuberculosis Commission to determine the prevalence of tuberculosis in the Saskatchewan population and to plan future sanatorium beds on the basis of the findings. Not only was his wish granted, but he was made secretary of the Commission when it was appointed by Order-in-Council on 22 July 1921, thereby gaining the staff and funds to research the extent of the TB problem in Saskatchewan. The recommendations of the final Commission report did not gather dust upon a shelf, as do many government reports today, but instead formulated Ferguson's lifelong objectives. Few medical men have had, early in their careers, an opportunity to document the extent of a target disease and in doing so, to plan for ways to combat it, setting the direction of their life work.

Of the Commission's recommendations, published in October 1922, the first four were considered mandatory:[8]

1 Hospital and sanatorium accommodation must be increased to care for those who are spreaders of the disease. The Commission recommended the construction of two new sanatoria of at least one hundred beds each, to allow the average patient twelve months of treatment.
2 There must be provision for the care of children from homes where open tuberculosis is found. A preventorium should be established to prevent the newborn infant from contracting tuberculosis from its mother. Children should be separated from actively tuberculous parents.
3 The system of financing the cost of treatment must enable all those who need treatment to obtain it with the least delay.
4 Diagnostic facilities must be improved and extended to all parts of the province, along with a nursing service and follow-up of all ex-tuberculous patients. Free diagnostic and follow-up clinics were set up in two Saskatoon hospitals and at Fort San.

As a further bonus, when the Commission disbanded Ferguson co-opted its chairman, A.B. Cook, Regina's sheriff, to become managing director of the Saskatchewan Anti-tuberculosis League and thus ensured its success.

First representative cross-sectional school studies (1921)
As part of the research necessary for the Commission report, arrangements were made with school boards to examine about 200 children between the ages of six and

fourteen in each of seven representative communities: Regina, Saskatoon, Moose Jaw, North Battleford, Cupar, Stoughton, and Heward. Each child received a physical examination by a chest specialist, an ear, nose, and throat specialist, and a dentist. Eighty of these children were selected, on the basis of physical findings, for a chest radiograph.[9]

Of the 1,184 children examined, 10 had active tuberculosis; another 15 were found to have tuberculosis on the follow-up chest radiograph. A positive tuberculin test in 56.6% of children indicated they had been exposed to tuberculosis (44% by age six and 61% by age fourteen). Of an additional 162 Indian children examined in residential schools, 93.1% had a positive tuberculin test.

Normal School students had a 75.6% positive tuberculin rate, and 0.9% had active tuberculosis. They were followed up annually throughout Ferguson's career; he watched with satisfaction the steady drop in the rate of positive tests.

Of 185 dairy cows in the same communities, 18.5% tested positive.

These baseline studies were, for their era, unusually sophisticated proportional samplings of representative communities. Wherrett confirms that they were the first in Canada.[10]

First traveling TB clinics, 1923
The Wherrett-Grzybowski report in May 1966 acknowledged that the credit for sponsoring Canada's first traveling clinics was shared between Saskatchewan and Ontario.[11] Clinics began in Regina in September 1923 and in Moose Jaw in May 1928, and for some years were held one day per week. Once-a-month clinics, chiefly for patients referred by general practitioners for diagnosis of lung disease, were held

in North Battleford and Swift Current (beginning in 1930), Yorkton and Canora (1933), Tisdale and Melfort (1934), and Wadena (1940).[12]

First universal free diagnosis and treatment of TB,
1 January 1929
Ferguson worked systematically to gain grassroots support for free treatment of tuberculosis, advocated in the Commission report in 1922. It took seven years.

Few could afford to pay for a year or more of treatment in a sanatorium. But from 1917 until 1928 it was Saskatchewan's policy that "all who were able to pay were required to pay." In 1924, 29 of 295 patients (9.8%) paid part of the costs for their treatment, even though some were bankrupted and returned home penniless. By 1928, only 2.5% could pay for their treatment. The other 97.5% required at least partial financial help from their urban or rural municipal government.

Saskatchewan's Rural Municipal Act of 1920 required each RM to contribute $100 annually to the sanatorium. In 1921, the $30,100 from 301 rural municipalities was set aside as the nucleus of a pool to pay for the treatment of indigent rural patients. Rural municipalities in this way got a four-year head start on their urban counterparts, on the path towards "free treatment."

The Saskatchewan Association of Rural Municipalities (SARM), then the most influential organization in the province, complained at its annual meeting in March 1921 that the urban municipalities were exempt from this levy. In 1925, an urban pool was formed. Without both rural and urban municipal contributions, the sanatoria would have been insolvent.

The first resolution to advocate totally free treatment for tuberculosis was introduced at the SARM annual meeting in 1925. Only six of the 600 representatives voted for it. Yet the seed had been planted and the idea grew. In 1926, there were twenty votes in favour. In 1927, a different motion, that the provincial government take over direct control of the sanatoria, carried by a small majority. The government, normally very responsive to resolutions from SARM, countered that they could not afford it.

At the annual meeting of SARM in March 1928, a momentous resolution was moved by RM Weyburn #67 to petition Saskatchewan legislators "to amend the Sanatoria Act so that all classes of T.B. patients shall have free treatment available at the public expense ... paid partly by the [provincial] government [and] partly by all rural and urban municipalities."[13]

In the midst of the discussion, an ex-patient of Fort Qu'Appelle Sanatorium, now cured and employed as secretary of his municipality for nine years, stood up. There, before the eyes of all doubting Thomases, as was remarked later, stood a living example of what could be and was being done through efficient and timely treatment of the tuberculous. This time the motion passed unanimously. A similar resolution was later passed by the Saskatchewan Urban Municipal Association and by the United Farmers.

Times were good just before the stock market crash and the depression. As soon as the legislature next met, early in December 1928, the Liberal government of James G. Gardiner presented the Saskatchewan Sanatoria and Hospitals Act. As a government bill, it passed readily. What was amazing was the speed of implementation. The new system of free treatment came into effect in less than a month, on

1 January 1929. The Honourable Sam J. Latta, minister of municipal affairs, characterized the new Act as "a great social experiment – and a costly one at that."[14] Roughly half of the League's operating funds came directly from the rural and urban municipalities, a greater participation than in any other province, "a distinctly Saskatchewan approach."[15] The municipal funding, of course, was not subject to competition from highways and welfare in annual government budgets. It was not unusual for a rural municipality in a given year to spend more money on one disease, tuberculosis, than on roads!

There were immediate benefits. As Ferguson reported, "the effect of removing the financial barrier is earlier treatment, earlier isolation, and an [initial] increase in the number of days treatment and the gross cost, but the end result will be more cures and a shorter period of disability, lessened spread of the disease, a lower death rate, and eventually [fewer] new cases."[16] It was seven years before the next province, Alberta, offered free treatment in 1936. Manitoba followed in 1946.

Saskatchewan's health minister, Allan Blakeney, said in 1964, "the introduction of diagnosis and treatment of tuberculosis at public expense was one of the early and essential steps in developing a program of health services available to all."[17] To have Saskatchewan lead all other jurisdictions in North America, the first to provide free treatment of tuberculosis, the most expensive disease that took longest to cure, was one of Ferguson's greatest accomplishments. Saskatchewan's success with universal availability of tuberculosis diagnosis and treatment became an important stepping stone toward universal hospitalization insurance and medicare.

Epidemiology: A landmark study of TB *among Indians*
(1928)

Ferguson's study of the prevalence of tuberculosis as it reached "fertile ground," a population with no previous history of exposure to the disease, is one of the best of a very few epidemiologic accounts of such a process anywhere in the world. A new infection, arriving for the first time, hits with great severity, affects almost any body organ at any age, and has a high mortality. Then, as the most susceptible die off and only the more resistant individuals survive, there is a natural and inevitable drop in the number of new cases of that disease.

It is more humane and more efficient to prevent disease than to cure it. With his deep concern for those we now term First Nations people, Ferguson obtained annual research grants from Canada's National Research Council (NRC), from 1926 until his retirement in 1948. These grants financed his studies of TB prevalence on adjacent Indian reserves, the first Bacille Calmette Guerin (BCG) vaccination of Indian infants, and the first in student nurses. The NRC had been formed on 29 November 1916, and its eleventh committee was formed in 1925 to study tuberculosis, initially in cattle.

Ferguson graphed the rapid increase in deaths from tuberculosis among Indians at the Qu'Appelle and File Hills agencies (Figure 4–3) as they settled in small houses in close proximity to each other on reserves. Under the new conditions of stationary life, intermittent hunger, and cultural demoralization, the annual Indian death rate from tuberculosis was roughly 1,000 per 100,000 population in 1881. It quickly increased to reach the proportions of a serious epidemic by 1884, and became maximal in 1886 at 9,000 per

100,000 per year, about double the birth rate and accounting for two-thirds of all Indian deaths. By 1895 the rate had dropped to 3,000, by 1901 to 2,000, and by 1907 was back to 1,000 per 100,000. Changes in living or sanitary conditions did not explain the drop. Ferguson recognized that this was the inevitable and natural course of a new epidemic. Virtually all Indian children were "tuberculized"; by the age of eleven to fifteen, over 96% had a positive tuberculin test.

His field work began in 1926 with a thorough examination of Indian children on the File Hills and Qu'Appelle reserves and those attending the Lebret and File Hills Indian schools. Such surveys became annual events.

Ferguson recognized the need to determine the prevalence of tuberculosis in adult Indians as well. How was he to get them together for chest radiographs far from electrical

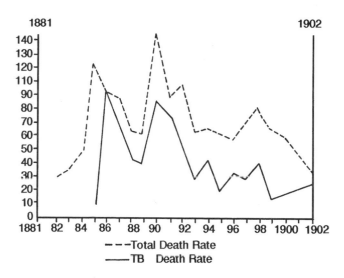

Figure 4–3 Graph of tuberculosis epidemic among Indians (SLA)

sources? He had the brilliant inspiration to join the annual treaty party, when all natives congregated to receive treaty money of $5 each. He persuaded the Victor X-ray Corporation of Winnipeg to supply a portable x-ray machine and the Delco Light Company of Regina to supply a portable generator. In the second week of July 1927, all this equipment accompanied the treaty party to the File Hills Reserve, where full compliance was achieved and 130 adult Indians were x-rayed.

In 1928, Ferguson presented his landmark report at the prestigious meeting of the National Association for the Prevention of Tuberculosis in Great Britain:

The moral and physical weakening of the Indian has to do with the introduction of the horse ... firearms ... liquor, the exchange of their fur tunics for the blanket, the exchange of the clothes necessary for warmth for alcohol, the extermination of the buffalo and the beaver, the concentrations upon reserves, the change of housing, the change of food, the exclusion of sun ... by the clothing of the children; the compulsory concentration of children in schools, the change of occupation from hunting and warring to agricultural pursuits, and, on the mental side, the psychical depression of conquest by the whites, dependence on Government rations for food, visible ravages of white man's diseases, desertion by, or incompetency of, their Michi-Manitou and triumph of Kitchi-Manitou, and failure of even the white man's religion to protect them ... The nudity of the Indian children in summer ... was ended abruptly ... The agents, in their zeal ... instructed the parents to clothe their children. Thus for the first time in the history of the race the bountiful summer sun's rays were largely excluded ... a lowering of resistance to disease developed."[18]

Ferguson's dedication to Indians is exemplified by the four-week canoe trip he took in 1927, departing from the end of steel at Big River, to inspect natives with tuberculosis at Ile-à-la-Crosse and La Loche. Six years later, Dr Andrews from the Prince Albert Sanatorium made the first airplane flight to Ile-à-la-Crosse.

Ferguson treated Indian patients as equals, as any compassionate doctor would. They in turn respected him. In 1935, they gave him what he considered the greatest honour of his life, a ceremony naming him as an honourary chief – Muskeke-O-Kemacan (Figure 4–4).

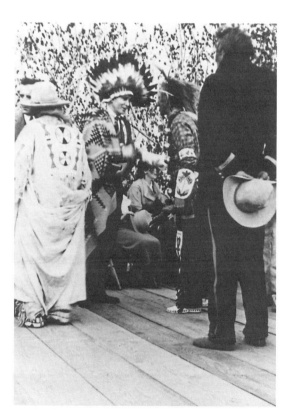

Figure 4–4
Muskeke-O-Kemacan,
Great White Physician
(SLA)

Indians were not legally a responsibility of the Saskatchewan Anti-tuberculosis League, a provincial organization, but of the Government of Canada. In spite of this, one of Ferguson's top priorities throughout his life was to reduce the ravages of the disease among Indians. He engineered an agreement with the federal government in 1924 whereby forty beds were allocated for Indians at the Sanatorium as a means of paying off some of the capital advanced to the province near the end of World War I. Once the Prince Albert Sanatorium opened on 7 January 1930, there were adequate beds for Indians, both adults and children. In striking contrast, Manitoba Indians gained access to sanatorium treatment only in 1946 when the Clearwater Sanatorium opened in wartime United States Air Force buildings.

First statistically controlled BCG vaccination among
newborn Indian infants, 1932–49
Between 1933 and 1943, Ferguson and his former University of Manitoba medical school classmate Dr Austin Simes, of the Indian Health Unit, vaccinated 306 Indian infants at birth. Another 303 infants served as controls. Their study was statistically sophisticated for its time – though through imperfect randomization by Dr Simes (tossing a coin for each subject would have been sufficient!), the BCG study lost the opportunity to be the world's first fully randomized clinical trial.[19] Ferguson and Simes' joint paper showed that the incidence of tuberculosis was nearly five times greater in the unvaccinated, whose disease was more severe and more widespread than in the vaccinated group.[20]

The BCG studies were carried out in the face of frank hostility to BCG throughout the English-speaking world, apart from the strong support of the Canadian BCG pioneer, Armand Frappier in Montreal. Other North American doctors mistrusted live-bacteria vaccines in general and BCG in particular.

First BCG vaccination among student nurses, 1934–43
Because 5% of student nurses and nurses in western Canadian hospitals "broke down" (the term used in standard medical parlance) with tuberculosis, all tuberculin-negative student nurses in Saskatchewan hospitals and all tuberculin-negative sanatorium and mental hospital employees were given BCG. Ferguson reported in 1946 that this measure reduced the number of cases of manifest tuberculosis to less than a quarter of the previous rate for nurses, to one-fifth of the previous rate for sanatorium employees, and to one-fifth of the rate among student nurses in adjoining Manitoba.[21] In subsequent years, this vaccination was extended to tuberculin-negative members of families in which tuberculosis had occurred.

First province-wide photofluorographic surveys, 1943–47
Ferguson organized the first province-wide photofluorographic survey in North America, 1943–47. Since no machines were available commercially, he encouraged his radiographer, Robert Connell (Figure 4–5), to develop a method of photographing a fluoroscopic screen with a 35 mm camera (Figure 4–6). Connell was aided by Richard Tizley, a welder hired on the day World War II began. A second-hand van was purchased for $250 and mobile community surveys began in 1941. The aim was to achieve early diagnosis, when the disease would respond most readily to the simple measures then available – bed rest, fresh air and

good food. During the second Saskatoon survey in 1948, 41,082 of the 43,016 residents were radiographed – the highest rate of participation ever reached (95.5%). About one new, active case of tuberculosis was found per thousand people.[22] The survey was staffed by unpaid local volunteers in each village or town, all vying for a higher turnout than the neighbouring town. Other expenses were met through funds raised by the ACT amateur hours on all Saskatchewan radio stations and by the annual Christmas Seal campaign. The survey of the entire province was completed in 1947; a second survey began immediately.

In 1948, the Anti-tuberculosis League began to pay for a chest radiograph of every patient admitted to hospital. This program was fully operative in every one of 109 Saskatchewan hospitals by 1950. Since people admitted to hospital were more apt to be ill, this became one of the most effective means of detecting new cases of tuberculosis and, as a side effect, detected a roughly equal number of unsuspected lung cancers.

First province with sufficient beds (three per TB death), 1942
From 1921 through 1940, Saskatchewan had a lower tuberculosis mortality rate than any other province.[23] Saskatchewan was the first province "to provide sufficient sanatorium beds to treat all tuberculous patients," the aimed-for ratio being three beds for every tuberculosis death.[24] The necessary facilities were disproportionate in size and cost for a poor province. High capital costs were combined with high costs of identifying patients with the disease.

Why was Saskatchewan a leader? The answer relates, in part, to the calibre of Ferguson, the strong support his own conviction generated, and the administration of the entire

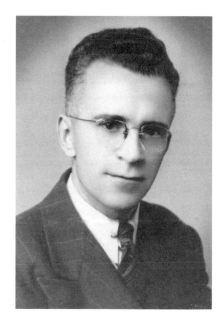

Figure 4–5
Robert Connell
(Mrs. G. Connell)

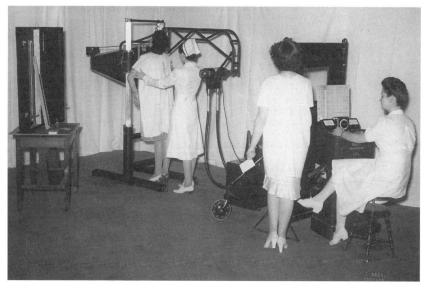

Figure 4–6 Photofluorograph machine used for mass TB surveys (SLA)

program by a "semi-official body, mainly lay and voluntary in its operation."[25] Where else could Ferguson have reached out to every farmer? Where else could he have garnered such solid grassroots support? Where else was such a highly developed social conscience and community co-operation the basis of everyday life? As Premier T.C. Douglas said at the 50th anniversary of the founding of the Anti-tuberculosis League, Saskatchewan people had developed "a special capacity to meet and solve problems that by far excels more fortunate places." Douglas was right. The League had obtained "the support and co-operation of the public to a greater degree than [in] any other province."[26] This public- spirited group has continued its work in preventive medicine since 1981 as the Saskatchewan Lung Association.[27]

Lowest tuberculosis death rate in Canada
Ferguson's work bore fruit. He witnessed the decline of case rates from 98/100,000 population in 1925 to 51/100,000 in 1948. However, incidence and death rates also declined in regions that lacked sanatoria, representing the natural course of any epidemic. Then, with the advent of streptomycin and para-amino-salicyclic acid in 1948, tuberculosis death rates fell sharply. The Prince Albert Sanatorium was closed in 1961, Fort San in 1972, and the Saskatoon San in 1981.

Ferguson in later life
Ferguson was made a Member of the Order of the British Empire (MBE) on the king's birthday in 1935. He received an honourary LLD from the University of Saskatchewan in 1946. He retired on his sixty-fifth birthday, 12 September 1948.

The next six years were spent in researching and writing his highly acclaimed book, *Studies in Tuberculosis*, published by the University of Toronto Press in 1955.[28] He received the prestigious Charles Mickle Fellowship in 1961. His portrait by artist Nicholas de Grandmaison was commissioned by his friends in 1962. Ferguson died on 1 March 1964.

Some reasons for Ferguson's success

Ferguson had the full support of the League's dedicated board of directors. Peter McAra was mayor of Regina when he became the founding president of the League; McAra continued on the board of directors after he stepped down as first president, and he served again as president from 1930 to 1941. E.G. Hingley represented SARM for forty years and was president of the League from 1945 until his death in 1958. Dr F.W. Hart of Indian Head, an original trustee from 1911 to 1918, returned to the board as representative of the Saskatchewan Medical Association from 1932 to 1946. His son, Bob, married Ferguson's daughter, Helen.

Ferguson's timing throughout the first thirteen years of his campaign was perfect. The return of veterans after World War I caused the federal government to pour needed money into new buildings at Fort San; the higher federal per diem rate also helped augment the League's bank balance. Free tuberculosis treatment passed the legislature in 1928, in part because the farm economy was buoyant in the late 1920s. World War I had also changed public attitudes more than anyone realized; few other "charities" had as much appeal.

All three Saskatchewan sanatoria took great care to maintain good relationships with all practising doctors. As Boughton said later of Ferguson, "One of his long suits was to play hand-in-glove with the doctors who referred patients."

Ferguson consistently gained maximum government support, yet he kept a tight rein on management. There was no patronage and no featherbedding. The League provided a marvellous bargain to Saskatchewan in terms of service per patient day per dollar. Whether the Liberals or Conservatives were in power, Ferguson had immediate access to the premier and the minister of public health. (When the CCF gained power, Tommy Douglas confided to my father that the province's recommendation to Ottawa that Ferguson be named Saskatchewan's lieutenant-governor had not been successful.)

The League, followed by the Saskatchewan Lung Association, operated the sanatoria and clinics – the entire tuberculosis program – until 1987. Members of each successive government realized, sometimes contrary to dogma, that the arrangement was mutually beneficial. The various levels of government put up the money, and the League ran the incredibly cost-efficient organization, with a great deal of help from many volunteers and private organizations. At the same time the League attracted exceptionally dedicated people and provided a high standard of care.

Ferguson's other appointments and awards included president of the Saskatchewan Medical Association (1922); fellow of the American College of Chest Physicians; member of the Senate of the University of Saskatchewan (1923–28); life member of the Royal Canadian Legion. R. G. Ferguson, MBE, BA, MD, LLD, 1883–1964, is remembered with respect and affection. His name is commemorated by the R.G. Ferguson professorship at the University of Saskatchewan, by the Dr George Ferguson School in Regina, and by one of Saskatchewan's largest islands, Ferguson Island in Montreal Lake. "His resting place is in the

valley he loved, but his shrine is in the hearts of the people
of Saskatchewan."[29]

George Ferguson! You should be here today.
Saskatchewan needs you: she believes that tuberculosis
Is controlled,
That public health is no longer at risk,
That the province's wealth should be used to acquire luxury.
Wake us up; show us again with your towering wisdom
How to walk the common path of man;
And perform the lowliest task with cheer.[30]

Postscript

The number of new cases of tuberculosis in Saskatchewan
non Indians decreased from 931 in 1926 to 43 in 1990. In
1962 the mobile x-ray took chest radiographs of 3,462 abo-
riginal people in northern Saskatchewan, those in the highest risk area, and found not one new case of TB. But the
apparent defeat of tuberculosis, especially in northern
Saskatchewan, was short-lived.

Sadly, the optimism so evident in 1964, the year Ferguson
died, has since palled. Saskatchewan is no longer a leader.
In 1987, its largest census area, the northern half of the
province, had the highest rate of active new cases of tuberculosis (248.6 per 100,000) of any complete census region
in Canada, and the Meadow Lake census division had the
eighth worst record in the country. Two Indian Reserves,
Buffalo River and Portage la Loche, had rates of 1,000 per
100,000, 400 times that of Caucasians in southern
Saskatchewan.[31]

In 1965, treaty Indians comprised 3% of the Saskatchewan population, yet they had 75 new (not previously

reported) cases of tuberculosis. These accounted for 34% of the provincial total, a rate of 260 per thousand. In 1990, Indians comprised 6% of the population; 156 new cases of tuberculosis accounted for 75% of the total, at a rate of 267 per thousand. In 1989, the proportion of patients with primary tuberculosis was 70% in Indians and only 5% in Caucasians, a striking difference.[32]

Directly Observed Therapy (DOT) was introduced into Saskatchewan in the autumn of 1989, to diminish the frequency of treatment failure and of very costly drug resistance. With another person identified to watch patients swallow their pills twice a week, selective breeding of resistant TB bacilli has greatly diminished.

In the first four years with DOT, compliance rose to over 85%, drug resistance diminished from 13% to 2%, costs decreased to one-fifth the amount for self-administered treatment, and there were fewer hospital admissions.[33]

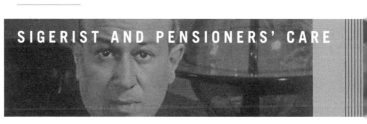

CHAPTER 5

SIGERIST AND PENSIONERS' CARE

North America's first social democratic government, 1944
"No person has had as profound an effect on the restructuring of health services in Canada as Tommy Douglas, that doughty little Scottish socialist fighter and orator"[1] (Figure 5–1). Douglas was "among the greatest political campaigners Canada has known."[2] His CCF party won a landslide victory, forty-three of the fifty-two seats, in the Saskatchewan election of 15 June 1944. Health was Tommy's number one priority then and throughout his tenure as premier.[3] To be certain that health matters were front and centre, Douglas assumed the health portfolio himself.[4] For his first four-year term of office and into his second term, he carried this heavy burden in addition to his responsibilities as premier.

The Sigerist Commission, 1944
One of Douglas's very first priorities, within two days of the election, was to contact Dr Henry Sigerist (Figure 5-2),

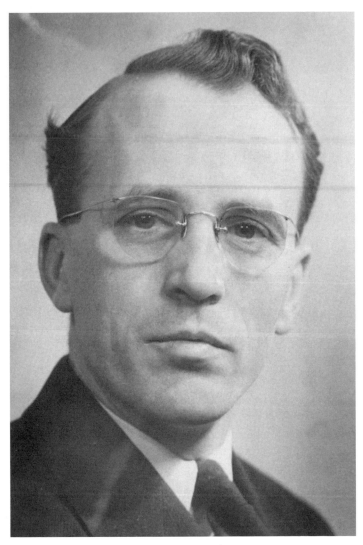

Figure 5–1 Premier T.C. Douglas (SAB R-A3421)

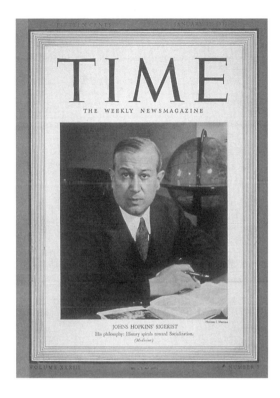

Figure 5–2
Henry Sigerist
(*Time Magazine* cover,
30 January 1939)

professor of the history of medicine at Johns Hopkins University,[5] and author of a book that took a rosy view of Soviet medicine,[6] to head a health study commission. Although Sigerist was a "physician of international reputation," as Malcolm Taylor wrote, "there was a great deal of criticism later that a professor of the history of medicine ... had been chosen rather than an expert in health services organization and administration."[7] Dr J. Lloyd Brown of Regina was the representative of the medical profession on the Sigerist Commission.[8]

Sigerist began work on 6 September 1944, completed visits and hearings on 23 September, finished the report at five minutes after midnight on 1 October,[9] and presented his formal report on 4 October.[10] As was the case with Lord Stephen Taylor, a medical doctor who gained the confidence of the profession and resolved the medicare dispute in 1962, Sigerist served without pay.

His stay in Saskatchewan was too short, yet he accomplished a great deal. He recommended establishment of district health regions for preventive medicine, each centred on a district hospital equipped with an x-ray machine, a medical laboratory, and an ambulance. He advocated rural health centres of eight to ten maternity beds, staffed by a registered nurse and one or more municipal doctors. The municipal doctor plans, he wrote, should be "maintained and developed."[11] He noted that the public must be educated to seek medical advice at the centre, so that each doctor would no longer "spend a large part of his time driving around the country."

Recognizing that municipal doctors were overworked and underpaid, Sigerist suggested that they receive annual vacations with pay. He proposed "free hospitalization," which he estimated would cost $3.60 per person per annum,[12] and would require another 1,000 to 1,500 hospital beds in Saskatchewan, including a 500-bed university hospital attached to a new medical college in Saskatoon. He analysed succinctly the then-current situation and offered solutions.

It is easy, with hindsight, to realize that Sigerist's crystal ball left much to be desired. His recommendation to build or improve many small village hospitals would have been appropriate in the 1930s but not as forward planning for the 1950s and 1960s. By following his report, Saskatchewan was saddled with too many small, one-doctor hospitals. Sigerist did not foresee that, farther down the road, the larger hospital with better facilities and two or more doctors could, with improved highways, be reached more quickly in subsequent decades. Nor did he realize that doctors would desire relief from being on call twenty-four hours a day, seven days a week.

Sigerist, a historian of medicine and not a futurist, also failed to foresee the rapidity of technological change that was already on the horizon. He overlooked the fact that larger farm machinery and highway improvement would contribute to rapid decline in the population of rural municipalities and villages and to increasing use by rural people of business and professional services in the cities. In the hospitals, rather than suggesting there be training of more x-ray technicians, or of combined laboratory and x-ray technologists appropriate for one-doctor hospitals, he recommended that "one nurse in every hospital be trained to handle the x-ray machine and the routine clinical laboratory work."[13] When he advocated consideration of sterilization for mental defectives, then popular in many jurisdictions, he failed to appreciate the ethical considerations involved. He demonstrated incredible naïveté when he prophesied that the complete eradication of venereal disease could be achieved in the near future.

Professor Milton Roemer of the University of California, Los Angeles, nonetheless described the Sigerist report as "one of the most advanced health services reports of its time."[14] It provided the "blueprint" for medical care in Saskatchewan for half a century. Sigerist, in looking back on his life in 1950, admitted that he had rarely experienced "a warm feeling of having accomplished a job well," but that one of these occasions was in 1944, on returning from Saskatchewan.[15]

Douglas's promises to doctors

At no time did Douglas make a salaried medical service a CCF platform plank.[16] Indeed, his letter to J. Lloyd Brown dated 19 September 1945, published in the *Saskatchewan Medical Quarterly* that December, promised the medical profession that: 1) "a health insurance scheme shall be administered by a Commission which shall be free from political interference and influence"; 2) this Commission "shall be representative of the public, those giving the service, and the Government"; 3) the Commission "shall have sufficient power and jurisdiction to establish and to administer a plan"; 4) the chairman "shall be a physician"; 5) "no commissioner, representing a profession, shall be appointed except with the approval of the profession concerned"; and 6) "the professional committees shall have unrestricted jurisdiction over all scientific, technical, and professional matters."[17]

First comprehensive health plan for pensioners and widows, 1945

Douglas's next urgent health priority was to provide comprehensive health care for those requiring social assistance, "old age and blind pensioners, widows on mother's allowance, and their dependents." There were 28,000 such people on the government rolls.[18] On average, each doctor would have about fifty of these people as patients.

Douglas met with the council of the College of Physicians and Surgeons of Saskatchewan on 23 August 1944. The profession co-operated to the fullest. My father came home from the meeting bemused by the course of events. Douglas had asked the council for their estimate of what such a program would cost. The doctors did not know. They asked Douglas for his best guess. He didn't know. Both sides recognized that these patients required an above-average amount of medical care. Nevertheless, they amicably agreed to use the figure suggested as the cost of medical care by the federal Heagerty Interdepartmental Advisory Committee on Health Insurance in December 1942 – $9.50 per person per year.[19] At the annual meeting of the Saskatchewan Medical Association in September 1944, doctors agreed to control and administer the plan for the agreed-upon fixed lump sum, on a one-year experimental basis. Final agreement was concluded on 1 October, for implementation on 1 January 1945.

This cordial agreement, reached "with extraordinary speed,"[20] was welcome to everyone – what we would call today a win-win decision. The patients gained the right to health care without incurring a debt they had little hope of paying. Their families were relieved of responsibility. Municipalities were freed from any obligation to pay for indigents' care. The doctors were paid for caring for individuals who had rarely been able to pay them in the past. The profession's cornerstone method of payment – fee-for-service – had not been challenged. The key benefit for the government side, lost in all subsequent financing of health care, was that it could budget for an exact sum, the "ceiling principle," without risk of over-expenditure.[21] Further, the government's right to fund a major medical care program had been acknowledged.[22] Douglas had achieved his first health goal and his government had scored on the public opinion front. This scenario was as close to perfection as was ever possible in an imperfect world. The scheme was a success.

The doctors themselves policed this scheme to ensure an equitable division of earnings. They could be much tougher on an over-billing member than any government agency. A doctor submitting an account was paid fifty cents on the dollar. The residual was divided proportionately at the end of the year, depending on the number of dollars unexpended in the fund. In 1945, the final payment brought that year's earnings to 77.5% of the fee schedule, and then in 1946, with increased utilization by patients, earnings dropped to 59%. That year each doctor received a cheque at the end of the year for the final 9%.[23] In 1949, the profession negotiated a raise to $12 per capita,[24] then to $15, and finally to $21 in 1958.[25]

The Sigerist report and the social assistance health plan were solid achievements in the first six months of North America's first socialist government. Douglas deserves full credit for giving health a higher priority than any political leader before or since. His dedication was coupled with charisma, a legendary sense of humour, and a remarkable adaptability which made the best of any situation. McLeod and McLeod note that Douglas had "brought to the political life of the country a civility that enriched the Canadian scene," while carrying "a remarkably light load of ideological dogma."[26]

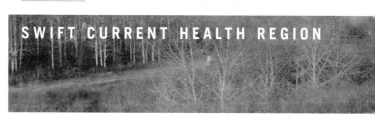

CHAPTER 6

SWIFT CURRENT HEALTH REGION

*First comprehensive health care and, for six months, the
first comprehensive hospital plan in North America, 1946.
First region in Canada to combine public health with
medical care, 1946*

Joan Feather opens her two landmark articles on the history of the Swift Current Health Region with the following
statement:

Southwestern Saskatchewan seems an unlikely place for a major
experiment in universal, prepaid health services. Rolling grass-
land, short, hardy crops struggling against drought and wind, vast
expanses without signs of human dwelling – how can such a place
give rise to a sophisticated service structure? The explanation is to
be found in the unique combination of past experience, local leadership, and government policy, skilfully merged into an experiment with remarkable staying power.[1]

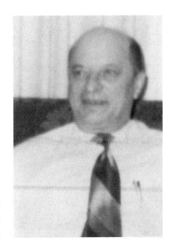

Figure 6–1
William J. Burak
(Mrs. Jean Burak)

Past experience and local leadership were exemplified especially by RM Pittville #169 at Hazlet. In 1939, Pittville paid Dr A.L. Caldwell of Cabri a municipal doctor salary of $2,700 per year; Pittville constituted less than half of his practice area.[2] When Caldwell joined the army in November 1941, the arrangement evolved so that residents paid a personal tax and carried a card that paid any doctor, anywhere in Saskatchewan, 50% of the fee schedule as payment in full, and paid any hospital $2.75 per day.[3] Pittville residents thus were not restricted to the services of a single salaried doctor, as was the case with municipal doctor plans. This freedom of choice was popular. In 1943, 1,200 Pittville residents were covered for a total cost of $13,031, or $10.91 per capita, a bargain for medical and hospital insurance combined.[4]

Pittville's secretary-treasurer, William J. Burak (Figure 6-1), was certain that his Pittville plan should be extended throughout the entire Southwest. In January 1945, he wrote to each municipality, proposing that they organize to form a health region to offer not just preventive medicine but a full health plan. The council of RM Pittville was the first to ask the government to establish a health region.[5]

A rather similar health plan had begun in RM Webb #138 under guidance of its secretary-treasurer, Stewart Robertson. It cost $7 per person or up to $50 per family.[6]

Swift Current needed a new hospital. In August 1945, Dr Mindel C. Sheps came from the year-old Health Services Planning Commission in Regina to discuss possible formation of a union hospital district.[7] Rather than have a separate meeting to discuss a health region, she suggested to Burak that "the question of organizing a health region could be discussed there."[8] As a spinoff from that meeting, Burak was appointed a committee of one "to sound out the surrounding municipalities." A veritable whirlwind, a "mover and shaker," as Lester Jorgenson called him,[9] Burak lost no time. He sent a four-page single- spaced mimeographed letter on 23 August and a follow-up three-page letter on 30 August to thirty-one rural municipalities, thirty-six villages, six towns, and the City of Swift Current,[10] offering his vision of a much larger enterprise, the formation of a region that would offer "complete medical, surgical and hospital services." Burak also took his personal crusade to the regional weekly newspapers[11] and attended regular council meetings of five rural municipalities to advance his proposals.[12] He then called a meeting, which he chaired on 15 September 1945; forty-eight of the invited municipal governments sent delegates. The other two members of Burak's organizing committee were Walter Melrose of RM Big Stick #141 at Golden Prairie and Carl Kjorven of RM Riverside #168 at Pennant.[13]

Premier Douglas had expressed doubt about the Swift Current priorities; he thought it prudent to have a slower evolution to full medical care. In a radio broadcast Douglas downplayed the necessity of a full regional plan.[14] In an article in the *Saskatchewan Medical Quarterly* in December 1955, Douglas wrote that he wished to introduce a health program, "step by step." He wrote of regional public health districts and hoped that "at least one public health district [would] be organized as soon as possible" – intending to begin with preventive services.[15] Joan Feather confirms this; the government had planned an experimental health region "with a focus on public health services and diagnostic and specialized facilities. But ... popular pressures forced a commitment to complete health services at public expense for the region."[16] Burak, who had given a lot of his time and spent his own money, never reimbursed, for "stamps, stationery, telephones, travelling and all other expenses,"[17] won out with his grandiose plan.[18] A vote was held in these municipalities on 26 November 1945.[19] The ballot read "Do you want a comprehensive system of health insurance, hospital and medical care and preventative services?"[20] By a 71% vote (Shaunavon's voters were barely in favour, 137 to 136),[21] the residents of southwestern Saskatchewan voted to establish a health region. The Douglas CCF government, to its credit, responded promptly to regional wishes. It passed an Order-in-Council on 11 December 1945 authorizing formation of Swift Current Health Region No. 1.[22]

On 17 January 1946, the organizational meeting, attended by sixty of the eligible eighty delegates, passed a simple resolution, "That the Regional Board of Health be instructed to provide hospital, medical, and limited dental care as soon as possible and that the funds required be raised by 25

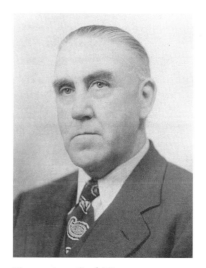

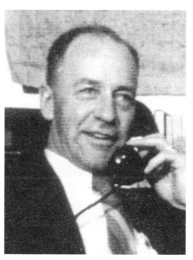

Figure 6–2 Carl Kjorven
(Lester Jorgenson)

Figure 6–3 Stewart Robertson
(Leah Robertson Koldingnes)

per cent from a land tax and 75 per cent from a personal tax."[23] Carl Kjorven was selected as chair (Figure 6-2), and Stewart Robertson as secretary-treasurer (Figure 6-3).[24] The representatives from the district medical society[25] met with the executive of the Regional board on 3 May 1946. They accepted payment at 75% of the Saskatchewan medical fee schedule, and agreed to have a meeting once a year between themselves and the board. Each side trusted the other. The meeting lasted only fifteen minutes.

Dr Arthur F.W. Peart, the district medical health officer, arrived in January 1946 and preventive work began on 1 May. Peart moved on after only nine months and was replaced by Dr Lloyd Davey.[26] Universal medical and hospital care came into force throughout Health Region No. 1 on 1 July 1946, exactly two years ahead of Great Britain's

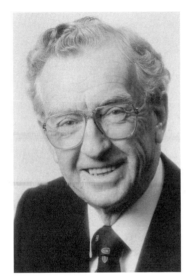

Figure 6–4
Dr Vince Matthews
(Pat Matthews)

National Health Insurance Plan, which began on 1 July 1948.[27] Dr Vincent L. Matthews (Figure 6-4), the third medical health officer, from 1 July 1948 through February 1957,[28] provided seamless integration of preventive work with medical care[29] and acted as accounts assessor and statistician for the Regional board. A man of integrity, Matthews quietly earned the respect of both the medical profession in the area and the general public.[30]

The drought-stricken Swift Current Health Region comprised an area of 13,932 square miles and a 1946 population of 53,597.[31] Only one year in approximately seven had provided a sound financial return to farmers. When the scheme began, only nineteen medical doctors resided in the Region, including four specialists in Swift Current.[32] With assured payment and, as doctors returned from service in the armed forces, increased availibility, the number of doctors jumped to thirty-four in 1947 and thirty-six in 1948. As Lloyd Brown reported: "a fine spirit of co-operation between the doctors and laymen on the Board was evident ... and a very evident desire ... to run their own affairs with a minimum of interference or control from the outside."[33]

The Region's staff, all paid by the Saskatchewan government, consisted of the medical health officer, seven public health nurses, a health educator, and three sanitary inspectors. Stewart Robertson, functioning as a chief executive officer, held this position until he retired at the end of 1966. Robertson was a frugal Scot who had left Scotland in 1920 at age twenty. Not only did he obtain full value for each dollar spent, but his own office was small, with second-hand furniture, bare wood floors, and no drapes. His first secretary, Pat Ditner, describes him as "caring, kind, sensitive, even-tempered, patient, compassionate ... hard working and willing."[34] Nothing flustered him. Each rural municipality and the city of Swift Current had an elected representative; all were laymen. Dr Orville Hjertaas of the Department of Health, assigned to organize health regions, remembered the "outstanding board of bright and caring people ... basically farmers."[35] The board contained "staunch Liberals and Conservatives and hard line C.C.F.ers, but they all left their politics on the doorstep."[36]

The Regional health scheme was financed by a personal tax – $15 for one person, $24 for two, $30 for three, and $35 for a family of four or more – and a property tax, calculated to raise 25% of the total, set at 2.2 mills. The provincial government contributed twenty-five cents per capita and paid one-half the cost of x-ray, dental, and outpatient services. The provincial contribution to the Swift Current plan in 1948 came to $63,691.[37] For the first six months of the scheme, hospitalization costs were 42% of total expenditures, having been underestimated by about $75,000.[38] Fortunately, the advent of province-wide universal hospitalization on 1 January 1947 saved the Swift Current plan from bankruptcy.

Expenditure for medical services within the Region, on a fee-for-service basis, was $410,453 in 1947 and $453,925 in 1948. In 1948, doctors received an average gross revenue of $12,880 – a net income averaging $8,114, since the overhead for a doctor in the area was estimated at 37%.[39] Referrals to specialists outside the Region, mainly Regina, came to $58,547 in 1947 and $67,909 in 1948. The per capita cost for medical service in 1947 was only $9.83 and in 1948, $10.23.[40] For the first time, as Dr J. Lloyd Brown pointed out, statisticians had access to reliable figures concerning the cost of medical care, a valuable side benefit from the operation of the Swift Current plan.

The Region's doctors were aware that specialists in Regina and Saskatoon looked askance at this experiment in "socialized medicine." Dr J.A. Matheson of Gull Lake said, "there have been times when we in the Swift Current area felt like black sheep ... We have been trying out some ideas that have not been approved." He went on to tell of the benefits of the scheme: "security and stability ... better incomes ... The patients are getting a better service ... partly due to an increase in the number of physicians."[41] Payment was in cash, no longer in chickens or sides of beef.

Dr Gordon Howden, a family practitioner in Maple Creek before he left to specialize in ophthalmology, gave a well-reasoned account of his experience. He found the scheme did not affect the doctor-patient relationship, but the doctor's work increased considerably and "many have acquired a taste for x-rays ... because of the good feeling and spirit of co-operation between ourselves and the Regional Board, we have had a excellent opportunity to present our case under favourable circumstances."[42]

One measure of success: the infant mortality rate is reputed to have fallen from a high level (before 1946) to the lowest rate in Saskatchewan in 1965 – 14.4 per thousand live births.[43]

Dr Arthur D. Kelly, deputy secretary of the Canadian Medical Association, visited the area in 1946. He found that the Regional board enjoyed "a large measure of local autonomy." He characterized the Region as "a successful experiment in the large-scale provision of medical care, courageously applied, efficiently managed and remarkably free from attempts to make the facts fit preconceived ideas, financial or otherwise."[44]

First regional hospital board in Canada, 1951
Vince Matthews' reminiscences include the information that the Swift Current Regional Hospital Council, formed in 1951, was the first regional hospital organization in Canada, an early precursor of a system that came into vogue, for better or for worse, in most Canadian provinces only in the 1980s and 1990s.[45]

As Maureen Matthews[46] said on her superlative CBC Ideas program with Lister Sinclair, 5 December 1990, "The basic idea was that every citizen deserved equal access to adequate medical care."[47] The following comments excerpted from that CBC program, provide the inside experience of two doctors in the scheme.

DR GORDON HOWDEN: The one thing that doctors and the municipal people felt ... was that it was our plan. It was a local plan, we could change things, we could communicate, there wasn't a political overtone at all. It was purely for the benefit of the people in the plan. ... the fact that it was on a small scale, the fact that it was a give-and-take situation with the municipalities and the doctors, both willing to learn, and being able to change the plans ... the doctors did feel that they had input.

DR CAS WOLAN: the Health Region trusted the doctors and the doctors trusted the Health Region ... after one of these meetings with Stewart Robertson for a few hours, we decided that for the balance of the year we'd go on fifty-one percent of our usual payments ... it was kind of a hard deal to take but I agreed to this thing, Stewart agreed to it, and I went back to the physicians and told them why and they accepted it.[48]

The secret of the Swift Current Health Region success was the integrity, pragmatism, and openness of all concerned. Dr Vince Matthews, Stewart Robertson, and Dr Cas Wolan, the doctors' representative for financial matters, would have coffee together most mornings at the Venice Café in Swift Current. If a new doctor to the area was over-servicing his patients or wanting to install an x-ray machine as a money-maker in his private office, the three would reach an amicable agreement to resolve the problem. Carl Kjorven, a farmer from near Cabri, was a skillful chairman.

Before the withdrawal of services of most Saskatchewan medical doctors in the still-remembered "doctors' strike" between 1 and 23 July 1962, the Swift Current Health

Region "asked to remain autonomous and carry on with their own successful plan."[49] But events became so emotional and so polarized that on 1 July the doctors within the Region closed their office doors in concert with those elsewhere in Saskatchewan.

After Lord Stephen Taylor's negotiated compromise on 23 July 1962, many doctors returned to work throughout Saskatchewan. The Swift Current area continued to operate separately from the provincial health plan, offering advantages over the rest of the province: no extra-billing and no hospital privilege problems.[50] An extra fee of $14 was added to pay for a children's dental plan. Collection of taxes and doctors' billings remained separate from the provincial plan.[51] In 1953, short of revenue, the Swift Current board added deterrent fees ($1 for an office visit and $2 for a house call).[52] By 1972, as part of a new federal-provincial agreement, the province assumed direct responsibility for medical services to those over 65, relieving the board of responsibility for this age group. By 1974, the Region ceased levying its own personal taxes. Until 1980, Regional cards continued to be issued annually by each RM and town office, but in 1981 the province moved the Region medical accounts into Regina.[53] Only in 1988 was the Region fully merged into the Saskatchewan Medical Care Insurance Commission, and the Swift Current office closed. The last Regional information meeting was held on 3 June 1993, the final vestige of local involvement.[54]

The Swift Current Health Region was a success. It was thoroughly tested. It was made to work. As Taylor says, "It had attracted a higher ratio of doctors-to-population than any other rural part of Saskatchewan."[55] The public, the doctors, and the inordinately small administrative staff felt a sense of ownership, of empowerment.[56] Swift Current became a major stepping stone on the road to medicare.[57] Lester Jorgenson of RM Miry Creek #229 emphasizes that this was a local, grassroots phenomenon. Although supported by the province, "the widely held concept that the Swift Current plan was a provincially directed pilot project does not fit the recorded facts."[58]

CHAPTER 7

MEDICAL COLLEGE
AND UNIVERSITY HOSPITAL

The success of any future medicare program in Saskatchewan required a first-rate medical school. Sigerist's report in 1944 recommended construction of a full, five-year medical school[1] and a 500-bed university hospital in Saskatoon. Sigerist predicted the building and equipping of the hospital and medical school would cost $2 million,[2] with annual operating costs of $150,000.

University of Saskatchewan medical college
Even before the 1944 election, T.C. Douglas planned a medical college when he took power. In thinking of possible candidates for a dean of medicine, he took advice from Dr W.C. Gibson, then serving at the Royal Canadian Air Force Clinical Investigation unit in Regina.[3] Gibson suggested his former teacher at McGill University, Dr J. Wendell Macleod.[4] However, it was not until July 1951 that the

provincial budget and Macleod's personal circumstances allowed him to accept the position. Macleod was a man of vision; he spent a year studying medical education and recruiting department heads before settling in Saskatoon.[5]

Meanwhile, in the spring of 1945, the legislature voted $100,000 to begin construction of the medical college; the cornerstone was laid by T.C. Douglas on 26 August 1946. The official opening took place on 8 May 1950.[6]

The first medical class was admitted in the fall of 1953 and graduated in 1958. There are benefits from a small class size. In spite of usually inadequate funding for the medical college, Saskatchewan medical graduates have done well. The history of the medical college has been chronicled through 1976 by Dr Douglas J. Buchan,[7] and from 1976 through 1998 by Dr Louis Horlick.[8]

University hospital
Premier Douglas established the Board of Governors for the university hospital in September 1946. In December 1946, he agreed to an expenditure of $7 million for a 550-bed hospital, to be connected to the medical building.[9] The legislature passed the University Hospital Act in 1947. Construction of three wings of the hospital began in 1948, but due to worrisome delays for financial reasons, the cornerstone was not laid by Premier Douglas until 19 September 1952. In his address, he wisely said "we wanted no medical school at all unless we could have the best possible."[10] The hospital opening ceremony took place on 14 May 1955.

Delays and inflation caused the price of the university hospital to rise far above the "ballpark estimate" of $1,500,000 given by Dr W.S. Lindsay, dean of the two-year basic science course in medicine, and adopted by Sigerist in his report. The final cost of the hospital was seven times higher – $10,589,703.[11] The university hospital brought top-notch specialists and subspecialists and greatly raised the standards of medical care in Saskatchewan, as recorded by Louis Horlick.[12] The medical college and university hospital were necessary ingredients in the preparation for medicare.

CHAPTER 8

PROVINCE-WIDE HOSPITALIZATION

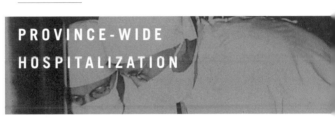

First province to provide capital grants for hospital construction, 1945

Saskatchewan took Sigerist's advice to heart in becoming the first province to provide funds for capital construction of hospitals, a major step on the road to medicare.[1] Between 16 March 1945 and 1 March 1949, the government provided $653,714 in outright construction grants and $173,500 in loans.[2] The National Health Grants Programme in 1948 added substantial federal funds to support hospital construction; Saskatchewan, sadly, having been too quick off the mark, was ineligible for matching federal funds for new construction since most of its hospitals had already been built. The province was in double jeopardy because some of the operational health programs had also been launched in anticipation of federal support; it was learned only too late that, because they were already underway, they were disqualified from receiving federal assistance.[3]

First universal hospitalization insurance program in
North America, 1 January 1947
Introduction of the first hospitalization insurance program
in North America was achieved in Saskatchewan with
remarkable speed and efficiency. Hospitalization was expected to cost even more than physician services and thus be
the most expensive "half" of the medicare equation.

Sigerist estimated that universal, province-wide hospitalization would cost $3.60 per person (about $3.5 million)[4]
per year and would require another 1,000 to 1,500 hospital
beds in Saskatchewan,[5] including a university hospital of at
least 500 beds.[6] The doctors in Saskatchewan enthusiasti-
cally and almost unanimously supported the introduction of
province-wide hospitalization on 1 January 1947. Doctors
could now admit patients to hospital whenever necessary,
without concern for cost.

Dr Mott and the Saskatchewan Health Services
Planning Commission
Dr Fred D. Mott (Figure 8–1), a graduate of McGill Medical School and a senior officer with the United States Public Health Service, became chairman of the Saskatchewan
Health Services Planning Commission on 1 September 1946.
Tommy Douglas deserves credit for making such a wise
choice. Mott's appointment was welcomed by the medical
profession, who viewed him as a big improvement in comparison to his predecessor.[7] Mott, a man of integrity and a
good listener, as well as a man of action, moved the plans
for the Saskatchewan Hospital Services Plan (SHSP) "into
high gear."[8]

The provincial hospital plan broke new ground. The administrative machinery had to be invented "from scratch,"

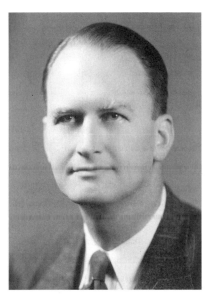

Figure 8–1
Dr Fred D. Mott
(SAB R-A7994)

and became the model for all subsequent plans. Malcolm Taylor, then an interested graduate student of health administration passing through Regina, describes the unprecedented pioneering effort as follows:

The new uniform hospital accounting system was finalized under G.W. Myers; the point system was completed,[9] the tax collection procedures agreed upon with the municipalities; and the organization of SHSP decided upon; scores of clerical, secretarial, and tabulating personnel were appointed and trained, and a massive publicity program was mounted to encourage early registration and tax payment.

It was a period of feverish activity, reminiscent of mobilization in 1939. The only office space available was in an ancient, vacated store building; clerical desks were long rows of plywood-on-trestles, with clerks sitting elbow-to-elbow, processing the registration and tax collection payments.[10]

The annual hospital premium was $5 for each adult and child, with a maximum of $30 per family. Each municipality received a 5% commission for collecting the premium. Patients no longer had to pay for in-patient hospital services.

The SHSP was administratively separate from the Department of Health but was not the "independent, non-political commission" the doctors had desired. The deputy minister of health sat on the commission, which oversaw both the SHSP and the Medical Services Division, which administered the Social Assistance Medical Care program (see chapter 5).

Sigerist's financial projections were wildly short of reality. The hospitalization costs for the first year were almost exactly twice his forecast – $7,560,763, a per capita cost of roughly $9.69. In subsequent years that $7.5 million seemed a bargain. Per capita costs of hospitalization rose rapidly, to $11.42 in 1948 and $13.59 in 1949. The most economical component in the early years was administration, which consumed only about 5% of total expenditures.[11] The $5 per person hospital tax initially covered 60% of the cost of province-wide hospitalization.[12] As Taylor says, "The tax collection system was successful to a degree unexpected for a regressive 'poll' tax." He adds, "In Saskatchewan, the plan became popular before it was expensive; in B.C., it was expensive before it was popular ... a main issue defeating the [British Columbia] government in 1952."[13]

Saskatchewan's immensely successful hospital insurance plan – the first in Canada – was introduced on schedule on 1 January 1947. By 1958, "the volume of hospital service received by Saskatchewan residents (2,100 days per 1,000 persons per year) was "the highest in North America ... their needs are being met."[14]

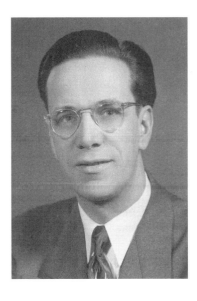

Figure 8–2
Malcolm G. Taylor
(SAB RWS-A11567, by
permission of copyright
holder Michael West)

The Saskatchewan Health Survey, 1949–51
A federal initiative to plan for medicare began on 28 July
1948, when the government of Canada announced that it
would make funds available for each province to survey
"present health services and facilities."[15] Saskatchewan
was allotted $43,506 for this purpose. A committee of
twelve had one representative each from registered nurses,
dentists, urban municipalities, rural municipalities, labour,
the hospital association, the farmers' union, the Swift Current Health Region (Carl Kjorven), and two from the medical association (C.J. Houston and G.G. Ferguson, registrar
of the Saskatchewan College of Physicians and Surgeons).
Dr Mott was chair and Malcolm G. Taylor (Figure 8–2)
was research director and secretary. The diverse group met
amicably;[16] as each question came up, it was hammered out

to the point of agreement. No minority report was submitted, nor were interim reports supplied to the organizations that each member represented. After more than two years' work and twenty-five meetings, the two-volume report contained a full catalogue of Saskatchewan's health resources and an estimate of needs in future.[17] Ken McTaggart felt this report surpassed that for any other province and described it as "the classic of such projects."[18] In addition, as C.J. Houston reported to the College of Physicians and Surgeons, the Saskatchewan committee "established a precedent in working out health matters. It has proved that a widely representative type of Commission can work."[19] Of 115 recommendations, the first was that "a comprehensive health insurance program should be undertaken at the earliest possible date."[20]

Hospitalization universal throughout Canada, 1961
British Columbia's hospitalization plan, the second in Canada, followed in 1949 but, lacking Saskatchewan's superb organization, suffered horrendous problems. On 1 January 1959, Ontario's plan went into effect. By 1961, all provinces were participating, but only after each had sent administrators to Regina to learn how to do it right. And cost-sharing by the federal government for 45% of the hospital plan, starting 1 July 1958,[21] now provided the Saskatchewan government with the funds it needed to undertake its long-sought goal of medicare.

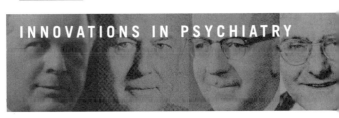

CHAPTER 9

INNOVATIONS IN PSYCHIATRY

When Saskatchewan became a province in 1905, psychiatry and mental hospitals across Canada were in a backwater compared to the rest of medicine. The first opportunity to show leadership was scuttled by unfortunate advice from Ontario.

A missed opportunity to pioneer small, humane psychiatric cottage hospitals, 1908

Dr David Low of Regina, the provincial health officer (Figure 9–1), was sent in 1907 to visit mental hospitals in eastern Canada and the United States. He was asked to consult widely and to make recommendations for construction of a mental hospital in the new province. He visited two up-to-date mental hospitals in New York State, at Ogdensburg and Ward Island, and the Protestant Hospital for the Insane at Verdun, Quebec. At these three hospitals, "instead of

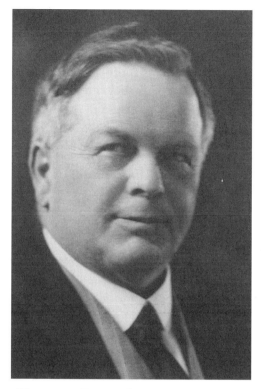

Figure 9–1 Dr David Low (SAB R-A3569)

measures of restraint such as padded cells and straight-jackets," there was sufficient staff and patients were allowed their freedom and even were allowed to use the libraries that were provided.[1]

Low recommended "a cottage system." However, Dr C.K. Clarke, superintendent of the Toronto Asylum, was asked to be a consultant to the Toronto architectural firm of Darling and Pearson, who were concerned about "scattered plumbing and heating lines" if a cottage plan were chosen. Clarke admitted that the cottage system is "ideal for the patients themselves, and provides means for breaking up the patients into smaller distinct groups," yet he advised against it on economic and climatic grounds.[2] It is a pity that the government chose to follow "expert advice" from Toronto and ignored Dr Low's recommendations. In retrospect, a series of cottages with closed-in connections between them, suitable for a cold climate, would have made Saskatchewan a leader, giving mentally ill patients more humane treatment at less expense. Sadly, the government opted for a more expensive pavilion-style institution at North Battleford,[3] which opened on 4 February 1914 with 314 patients. The patient population increased to 853 in 1920 and 985 in 1930. A second pavilion institution opened in Weyburn in 1921; it had 1,058 patients in 1930 and about 1,500 in 1963.[4]

Large mental hospitals were inherently counterproductive. "Patients came from long distances, tended to stay a long time and fairly often were not discharged. Deaths were high."[5] "The huge corridors and indefinite spaces would clearly be extremely damaging to people whose perceptual apparatus was already out of gear ... the large overcrowded institution not only did not help patients, it hurt them."[6]

First 500-hour psychiatric nurse training program in Canada, 1947

Dr Sam Lawson (Figure 9-2) wished to upgrade the attendants in the Saskatchewan Hospital, Weyburn. He devised a 500-hour program, one or two hours of lectures each day from October to June, to provide more expert and more humane care, and to upgrade the status of the caregivers.[7] A Registered Psychiatric Nurse (RPN) diploma was given to those who completed the course successfully.[8]

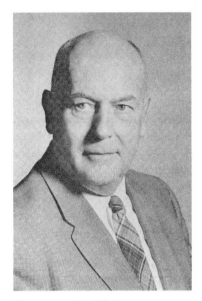

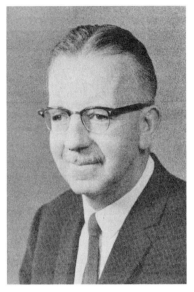

Figure 9–2 Dr F.S. Lawson
(SDCMH)

Figure 9–3 Dr D. Griffith
McKerracher (University of
Saskatchewan Archives)

First open psychiatric ward that included psychotic
patients in a general teaching hospital in Canada, 1955
When the university hospital opened its doors in 1955 in
Saskatoon, patients were treated almost exactly as were those
on medical and surgical wards, being free to visit the cafeteria and obtain passes to visit outside the hospital. Windows
were not barred. No one was restrained. From 660 admissions, patients left the ward without permission on seventy-
seven occasions; forty-four returned of their own accord,
fifteen were returned by relatives, eight by police, and six by
hospital staff.[9] The professor and head, Dr D. Griffith
McKerracher (Figure 9–3), even admitted ninety unselected
patients who had been committed to the Saskatchewan

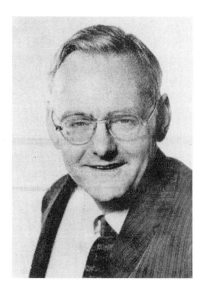

Figure 9–4
Dr Humphrey Osmond
(SDCMH)

Hospital at North Battleford and concluded that almost all mentally ill patients can be treated in a general hospital.[10] Family practitioners could visit their patients and some could take part in their care. The average length of stay was twenty-one days,[11] much shorter than the average stay (18.2 years, often until death!) at North Battleford.[12]

The Saskatchewan Plan, a first in Canada, 1956

In 1956, Dr Sam Lawson and K. Izumi, his architect, boldly presented their theoretical and unproven plan, named "The Saskatchewan Plan," to a meeting of the American Psychiatric Association Mental Hospital Institute in Denver, Colorado.[13] Dr John Mills[14] believes that doctors Sam Lawson, Griffith McKerracher, and Humphrey Osmond (Figure 9–4), the three senior psychiatrists at Weyburn, developed the plan through study and many long discussions, during the year or two before McKerracher accepted the headship of psychiatry at the new medical college in Saskatoon. The Saskatchewan Plan hoped to keep patients closer to their families through building eight or more small regional cottage hospitals designed by Izumi. Lawson expected that construction of the first regional cottage hospital, a radical departure in function and architecture and designed to "give the patients living conditions that are as near those of domestic living as possible,"[15] would begin in Swift Current in 1957, but it was delayed by four years and was then built in Yorkton instead.[16]

In striking contrast to the jail-like treatment in North American mental hospitals with large wards, where some patients were naked and others were kept in restraint, operation would be governed by the following six principles:

1 No human being should be incarcerated in an institution when any better solution can be found.
2 The mentally ill should have an equal standard of care to that given to the physically ill.
3 The continuity of care which is provided to the physically ill should also be provided to the mentally ill.
4 There should be integration of psychiatric care with general medical and surgical care.
5 Comprehensive care in the patient's home area should be made available.
6 In-patient facilities should be designed in such a way that they assist the patient's recovery.[17]

The key to the Saskatchewan Plan, as enunciated by McKerracher, was "community service, especially follow-up ... through a home-care program."[18]

First psychiatric ward to invite a general practitioner to treat (his) own mentally ill patients, 1957

Dr Abe Voth was the first (1957) and Dr Wilf McCorkell (1958 through 1 July 1961) the second family practitioner allotted two beds on the psychiatric ward of the new university hospital in Saskatoon.[19] Each had an interest in mental illness, attended psychiatric teaching rounds, and was asked by other family practitioners to see their patients. McKerracher said that McCorkell "participates in teaching with unusual success."[20] McCorkell published his experiences in treating sixty-four psychiatric patients.[21] His patients were discharged in an average of twenty-one days, although twenty-one of the sixty-four returned for further treatment.[22] Both Voth and McCorkell, from their contact and training, became more confident in dealing with mental patients in subsequent office practice.[23]

CHAPTER 10

HIGH-VOLTAGE CANCER TREATMENT

Saskatchewan was slow off the mark in using radiation to treat cancer but, once up to speed, it led the world. As with the initial provision of radium in 1932, high-voltage treatment could be available only with government support.

In 1922, Dr Ellice McDonald,[1] a Saskatchewan man who had been raised at Fort Qu'Appelle[2] and later specialized in cancer research at the University of Pennsylvania, visited University of Saskatchewan president Dr Walter Murray. McDonald informed Murray that the province of Quebec had just purchased a gram of radium for $75,000 and suggested that Saskatchewan should take similar action. In response, Murray wrote to Saskatchewan Premier Charles A. Dunning on 6 October 1922 to offer the services of university physicists if the province should decide to follow Quebec's example and offer cancer treatment to its citizens.[3] Dunning replied that the province's higher health priority was tuberculosis.[4]

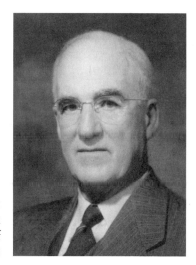

Figure 10–1
Dr Ertle L. Harrington
(University of
Saskatchewan Archives)

First cancer control agency in Canada, 1930
In 1929, the Saskatchewan Medical Association formed a
Cancer Committee; they enlisted Dr E.L. Harrington (Figure 10–1), professor of physics at the University of Saskatchewan, as their only non-medical member.⁵ Harrington's
advice led to the drafting of the Saskatchewan Cancer Commission Act, passed by the Conservative government of
J.T.M. Anderson in 1930.⁶ This act established the first cancer control agency in Canada and probably the first in
North America.

First government-sponsored cancer clinics in
North America, 1930
North America's first government-sponsored, part-time
(two mornings a week) consultative, diagnostic, and treatment clinics were staffed by radiologists: Dr Earle E. Shepley (Figure 10–2) at the Saskatoon City Hospital (beginning

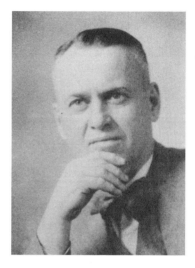

Figure 10–2
Dr Earle E. Shepley
(A. Becker)

in 1931),[7] and Dr Clarence M. Henry at the Regina General Hospital (1932).[8] Patients were treated with what were then called "high-voltage" machines, operating at 400 kilovolts peak.[9] Treatment and hospitalization were the financial responsibility of the patient,[10] but the government funded the equipment.

In 1931, Dr Shepley visited the leading cancer centres, particularly the Cancer Institute in Philadelphia, operated by Ellice McDonald, and the New York Memorial Hospital, under Dr James Ewing. On his return, Shepley submitted to the Saskatchewan Cancer Commission a thoughtful document, "The Essentials of an Ideal Cancer Policy."[11]

The Saskatchewan government allocated $115,000 for the purchase of radium in 1931.[12] From the university, Dr Harrington distributed radon to each of the cancer clinics in small gold tubes or "seeds" which had a 3.8-day half-life. Harrington was a proficient and enthusiastic glass-blower

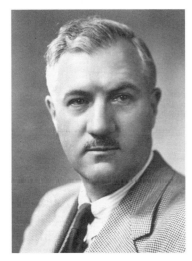

Figure 10–3
Dr Allan W. Blair
(SAB R-B11015)

who built and operated the radon plant from 1931 until 1962, extracting the radioactive gas emitted by radium in solution.[13]

The average number of patients referred per year to the two clinics increased, from 575 to 735 to 1,065, in the first four three-year periods until the end of 1943. In 1939, Dr Allan W. Blair (Figure 10–3), a Regina boy, a graduate of McGill University, and a radiotherapist at the Toronto General Hospital, took over as director of the Regina cancer clinic.[14]

Before the ninth legislature prorogued on 1 April 1944, the Liberal government of W.J. Patterson, under pressure from Dr George Dragan, who had been a backbench Liberal member from Kelvington in the eighth legislature, proclaimed a bare-bones cancer act, An Act Respecting the Control and Treatment of Cancer.

First in North America: Saskatchewan's Cancer Control Act, 1944

Following the CCF landslide victory on 15 June 1944, T.C. Douglas lost no time. Dr Blair was promoted to director of cancer services for the province; he served in this capacity until his sudden and untimely death from a heart attack on 9 November 1948. The first session of the legislature began on 19 October and ended on 10 November 1944. High on the Douglas agenda was the Cancer Control Act, which passed in October. Any person who had resided in the province for three months was now eligible for all services necessary for the diagnosis and treatment of cancer, without charge.[15] The program was paid entirely from government revenues. With free treatment, between 1944 and 1946 the number of patients jumped twofold to reach 2,626 in 1946.[16]

Canada's first full-time cancer physicist, Harold Johns, 1945

Blair was extremely foresighted in his recognition that the radiation treatment program would benefit from a full-time radiation physicist. Blair's first letter, dated 12 December 1944, to Dr Harrington at the university, suggested that a full-time physicist be hired jointly by the Saskatchewan Cancer Commission and the university. Six days later, Harrington replied, offering full co-operation. On 25 March 1945, Harrington hired Dr Harold E. Johns (Figure 10–4) for this joint position, with the rank of assistant professor, at $3,600 per annum. Johns was a thirty-year-old instructor at the Radar School at the University of Alberta, working for Canada's war effort. He had received his bachelor's degree in

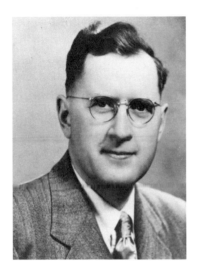

Figure 10–4
Dr Harold E. Johns (SCA)

physics from McMaster University in 1936, his master's from the University of Toronto in 1937 and his PhD from Toronto in 1939.[17] In his previous work at Edmonton Johns had used a radium source to obtain industrial photographs of steel propeller shafts to search for metal fatigue, a very early example of industrial radiography. In Saskatchewan, he was to give "half his time to supervision of the radium and x-ray therapy equipment of the two cancer clinics." Johns later told Lauriston Taylor that he thus became Canada's first full-time cancer physicist.[18]

In May 1946, Johns was given a travelling scholarship of $800,[19] which allowed him to visit, by train, the leading radiation physics centres in Canada and the United States. While in Toronto, he attended a series of lectures from Professor M.V. Mayneord, a senior medical physicist from the Royal Cancer Hospital in London, England. Mayneord, probably the first to do so, mentioned the possibility of using cobalt-60 as a radiation source. Harrington picked up on the idea; the next year in his presidential address to the Chemical, Mathematical and Physical Sciences Division of the Royal Society of Canada, he predicted that cobalt-60 "may become a more suitable source than radium itself in the treatment of cancer."[20]

Meanwhile, Johns returned home in 1946 with the conviction that another type of high-energy radiation source under development, the betatron, offered immediate promise. With Blair's support, Johns asked for a betatron of perhaps 35-MeV. The first 2.3-MeV betatron had been built in 1949 by Dr D.W. Kerst at the University of Illinois in Urbana and a 20-MeV prototype had then been built in 1942, based on the preliminary work of Dr Lester Skaggs.

University of Saskatchewan president James S. Thomson wrote to Blair on 18 November 1946: "I called last week upon Dr C.J. Mackenzie, President of the National Research Council, to discuss with him the use of a betatron in connection with the cancer treatment in this province. Dr MacKenzie ... expressed some doubts as to whether research was fully advanced to make such a project practicable ... Matters affecting the use of atomic energy are really under the control of the Atomic Energy Commission of which General A.G.L. McNaughton is the chairman." It did not hurt the cause that McNaughton was a native of Moosomin, Saskatchewan.[21]

Blair's reassuring letter to Mackenzie on 11 December 1946 was the cornerstone of all future developmental research in radiation therapy, followed consistently thereafter: "It is not planned to use it for any actual treatment until the physical measurements have been completed to everyone's satisfaction." This time-consuming attention to fine detail by Saskatoon physicists allowed those in another province, without such scruples, to, five years later, be the first to treat a patient with cobalt-60.

Meanwhile, other centres viewed the progress in Saskatchewan with suspicion. Harrington indicated their concerns in a letter to President Thomson on 20 February 1947:

In the earliest part of the discussion regarding the betatron, it appeared that a certain member of the Atomic Energy Commission, to which this matter must be referred for decision, had expressed the belief that if the reason for the betatron was mainly medical it would be in the interest of the country as a whole to locate it in a large medical centre, say, in Toronto. In the mind of Dean Mackenzie, the chance of obtaining a favourable action on our request for this equipment would be better if any possible uses in medicine of the betatron were given but little emphasis.[22]

The price tag for the betatron was high – $80,000. The Atomic Energy Control Board provided $30,000. Johns was disturbed because this amount was insufficient, but Blair was jubilant. "Spend that money, Johns," he said, "When it is gone more will be found."[23]

First concerted clinical use of the betatron in the world, 1949
On 3 May 1948, Johns, accompanied by Drs R.N.H. Haslam and L. Katz of the physics department, arrived in Milwaukee to examine "their" betatron. Where else could an agricultural province have found a manufacturer of heavy duty machines more suitable than an agricultural equipment company, in this case, Allis-Chalmers in Milwaukee, Wisconsin? Johns wrote back to Blair on 12 May 1948:

The betatron is finished but has not been tested. The machine which we are getting is the one ordered by the University of Pennsylvania, but they have no building finished to house it and have allowed us to have it. ... Professor Kerst has been more than cooperative. First he introduced us to all his men and gave us full access to *all* blueprints, *all* reprints, keys to the building ... Kerst then presented us with two donuts [sic] for nothing and one electron donut for a nominal sum ... Kerst is amazed at the rapidity with which we have pursued our program and in the fact we are getting the first betatron to be installed in any university or hospital ... The University of Illinois medical school gets the third betatron (second to the University of Pennsylvania) and I heard yesterday that the University of California is getting one, at Berkeley.[24]

The 24-MeV betatron was installed in the physics department at the University of Saskatchewan that summer (Figure 10–5). In keeping with the earlier promise, nine months were spent in meticulous calibration of this machine.[25] The

Figure 10–5 Betatron (SCA)

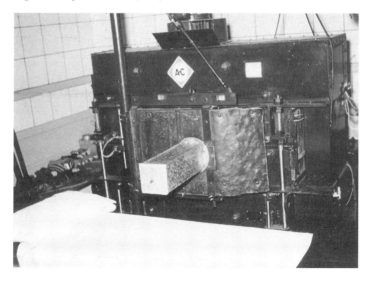

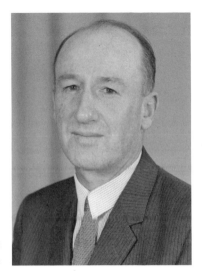

Figure 10–6
Dr T.A. Watson (SCA)

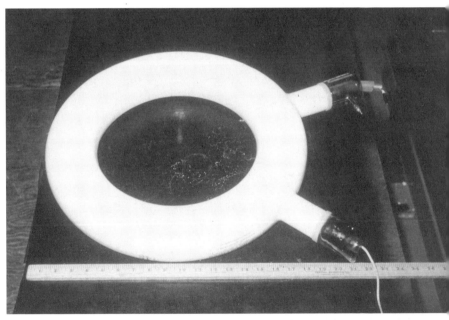

Figure 10–7 High-energy tube or "doughnut" (SCA)

first patient was treated on 29 March 1949. As Milford D. Schultz said of this Saskatoon machine in his historical review in 1975, "Thus started the really first concerted clinical investigation of the usefulness of multimegavoltage as a radiotherapeutic tool."[26]

The location of the betatron, in the physics department on the university campus, meant that patients were brought across the river from Saskatoon City Hospital and then across the campus. Even after University Hospital was completed on campus in 1955, there were still difficulties in transporting patients outdoors for a distance equivalent to several city blocks. The operating costs of the betatron were also exorbitant. Dr T.A. Watson (Figure 10–6), head of radiation oncology at the University of Saskatchewan, reported on 10 November 1949 to Dr O.H. Warwick of the National Cancer Institute that each betatron tube or "doughnut" cost $3,800 (Figure 10–7). Although "guaranteed" to last for 150 hours, "No doughnut which has so far been used has lasted nearly as long as this ... [T]he cost of the doughnut alone is $25.70 an hour ... eleven patients were treated at an average cost of $224 per patient." In seventeen years, only 301 patients were treated with the betatron.[27]

Nevertheless, as with any high energy source, the betatron offered "a method of delivering easily a high dose to tumours at a depth, without appreciably affecting the overlying skin ... Radiation sickness and blood changes are much less likely."[28]

First use of calibrated cobalt-60 in the world, 1951
In June 1949, Johns, keen to develop cobalt-60 as a more economical source of high-energy radiation, visited the Chalk River reactor in Ontario, the only installation in the world

then capable of producing large quantities of radioactive cobalt. There he visited with Drs A.J. Cipriani and W.B. Lewis of the Atomic Energy Project.

On 15 July 1949 Johns wrote to University of Saskatchewan President Walter P. Thompson, asking for an effective source of 1,000 curies of cobalt-60, about 100 times the activity of any radium unit. Johns asked for "between $2500 and $7000 to cover the total cost of construction." Johns, Cipriani, and Lewis agreed that this project would receive greater priority if it were considered as a research project, not a cancer treatment project. After a timely, quick visit to Premier and Health Minister Douglas in Regina,[29] to obtain his assent (see Introduction), Saskatchewan's simple two-page, three-copy application for the isotope was sent to the National Research Council at Chalk River on 13 August 1949.[30] It was a timely application. Three radioactive cobalt sources were placed in the Chalk River pile to "cook" in the fall of 1949.[31]

Saskatchewan received Chalk River's first cobalt source on 30 July 1951 and the University of Western Ontario received its source on 16 October of that year. These dates are of crucial importance, as will become evident. The third source was released for use in the United States in 1952.

Each cobalt source was 2.5 cm in diameter and 1.25 cm thick. Sybil Johns, Harold's wife, later described these as "a little half-inch stack of these cobalt discs about the size of a quarter."[32] As Johns had forecast, the approximate strength was 1,000 curies, or 37GBq. The Saskatoon unit was designed by Johns and Lloyd Bates, a graduate student, and was built by Johnny MacKay, the proprietor of Acme Machine and Electric in Saskatoon. It was installed in

Room 167 in the newly constructed cancer wing of University Hospital, adjacent to the medical college, on 17 August 1951. The room was hardly ready for use: the walls were still being plastered and the concrete floor had not yet been poured. Rigorous depth-dose measurements, using phantoms, soon began.[33]

The unit, weighing approximately 0.9 tonnes, consisted of a steel-encased cylinder suspended from an overhead carriage. A rotating, circular platform, flush with the floor, permitted rotation therapy (Figure 10–8). A variety of treatment fields could be obtained by using interchangeable lead plugs, developed and manufactured by MacKay. In order to turn the machine on and off, Johns and MacKay in essence reinvented the wheel (Figure 10–9). The radioactive cobalt source was mounted on the circumference of a wheel near the centre of the head. By rotating the wheel, the source could be moved 180 degrees from its shielded resting position until it was opposite an opening through which the radiation emerged.[34]

The *Saskatoon Star-Phoenix* on 18 August 1951 printed a photograph of the installation (Figure 10–10). The Saskatoon unit was officially commissioned on 23 October, but even more rigorous measurements were continued until 8 November, when the first patient was treated by Watson. Watson modestly but sincerely downplayed attempts to publicize the importance or the priority of Saskatoon's achievement, saying this was "merely a device that might provide more efficient and economical cancer treatment."[35] Steadfast to scientific integrity, being first was not important to any of the Saskatoon players, whereas London seems to have viewed it as a race to be won at almost any cost.

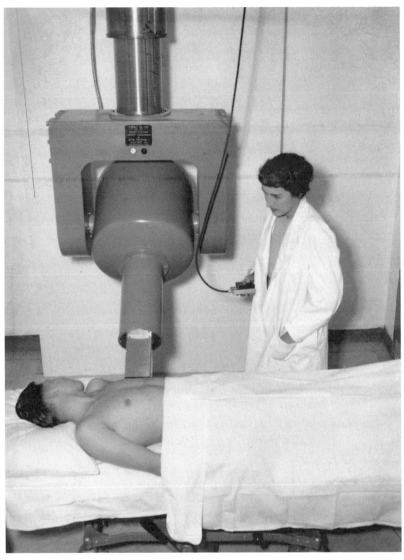

Figure 10–8 Cobalt-60 unit with Sylvia O. Fedoruk (SCA)

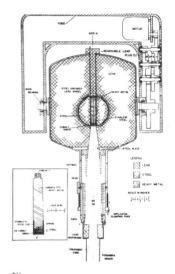

Figure 10-9
Diagram of cobalt-60 (SCA)

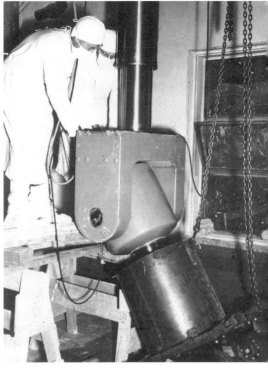

Figure 10–10 Installation of cobalt-60
(SCA and *Saskatoon Star-Phoenix*)

Eldorado Mining and Refining had completed the second unit for installation at Victoria Hospital in London, Ontario, on 23 October. Their unit, using a somewhat different design, consisted of a head pivoted between the arms of the horizontal "Y" that could be raised and lowered. The beam was turned on and off when a pool of mercury was introduced between the source and a conical opening in the head. The field size was varied by means of four lead blocks at right angles to each other. This was the prototype of the Atomic Energy of Canada Limited (AECL) cobalt unit.[36] Dr Ivan H. Smith quickly treated the first patient in London, Ontario, on 27 October, four days after installation.

The first cobalt treatment at London was widely publicized in the Canadian press. The *Saskatoon Star-Phoenix* commented on the "cobalt race" in an editorial on 7 November 1951:

We hope Messrs Truman, Stalin, Peron, et al won't think someone is trying to steal their thunder, but we think they ought to know theirs is not the only atomic race going on in the world. Another has been declared by *The London Free Press* which claims, editorially, 'the world's first cobalt bomb' for ... the Ontario city. With all due respect to the preservation of national peace and goodwill, that is a boast which this newspaper cannot allow to go unchallenged – especially since the *Free Press* reports that 'one is also being installed at Saskatoon, Sask.' One is indeed. Or, to be more accurate, one has been installed.

Historians can assess the relative merits of the two claims (Table 1). Suffice it to say that the first patient at London was treated with a machine that had not been calibrated. The patient had no hope of cure and died soon afterwards. The first patient at Saskatoon had advanced carcinoma of the cervix at age forty, unlikely to be cured by any treatment regimen then known. She received a precise dose to an exact area, carefully calibrated. Not only was she cured of her cancer, but she lived to the advanced age of ninety years in Victoria, British Columbia. She died on 26 October 1998.[37]

London was first in the public relations competition, but would its methodology have passed an ethics committee? In retrospect, one might question the ethics of "treating" a patient with an approximate dose of radiation to an approximate area of her body, with an uncalibrated machine, and with little hope for palliation, much less cure. The Saskatoon

Table 1
The first cobalt-60 treatments in the world, 1951

Saskatchewan	W. Ontario	
Cobalt-60 source delivered	30 July	16 October
Unit installed	17 August	23 October
Calibration	11 weeks	–
First patient treated	8 November	27 October

group may have come out second in boasting to the public, but they were first in achievement and in promulgation of their results to the scientific world.

The first formal publication giving details of cobalt therapy was from Saskatoon, not London. It was brief and to the point, much as Wilhelm Carl von Röntgen's first published description of x-rays had been fifty-four years earlier.[38] The authors of the report from Saskatoon, sometimes referred to privately and affectionately as the "Saskatchewan mafia," were H.E. Johns, L.M. Bates, E.R. Epp, D.V. Cormack, and S.O. Fedoruk, all from Saskatchewan, and three University of Saskatchewan physics graduates (A. Morrison, W.R. Dixon, and C. Garrett), working at the radiology laboratory in the physics division of the National Research Council in Ottawa. Their paper describes both Canadian cobalt units and concludes, "The cobalt units are flexible, simple to operate, and should require little servicing. They may prove to be very convenient sources of high-energy radiation."[39] A second paper by the same authors appeared in *Science* in March 1952.[40] More detailed papers on the calibration and use of the two units and the Saskatchewan betatron filled an entire issue of the *Journal*

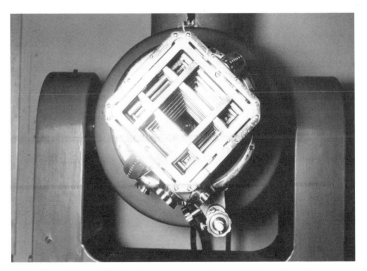

Figure 10–11 Collimation apparatus for cobalt-60 (SCA)

of the Canadian Association of Radiologists in March 1952. The Saskatchewan cobalt-60 depth-dose data[41] were included in a regular issue and a special supplement to the *British Journal of Radiology* in 1951 and 1952. Additional Saskatoon contributions to dosimetry appeared in other American, British, and Swedish radiology journals. The depth-dose charts compiled by Fedoruk and Johns were on the walls of active radiotherapy departments throughout the world.

MacKay turned his attention to designing a new collimator system, whereby a large number of interleaved diaphragms replaced the lead plugs, to direct the rays precisely (Figure 10–11). MacKay's small engineering firm in Saskatoon produced these collimators for over 100 Picker Cobalt units that were distributed around the world. The original

Saskatoon cobalt-60 unit treated 6,728 patients over twenty-one years until finally it was replaced by a commercial AECL cobalt-60 machine in 1972. Since the cobalt-60 unit was compact and economical to purchase and maintain, it became the "workhorse" for high-voltage radiotherapy for thirty years. By 1984, there were about 2,500 cobalt-60 units in routine use in the free world, 1,500 of which had been built in Canada by AECL.[42] These machines remain the only affordable radiotherapy option in many third world countries.

As Sylvia Fedoruk and I wrote in our chapter in the book produced to celebrate the 100th anniversary of Röntgen's discovery of the x-ray: "Though born of war-time nuclear research, the cobalt bomb was in practice a ploughshare rather than a sword, and a largely Canadian contribution to medical care. With its flair for trend-setting performance in medicine, Saskatchewan had led the way."[43]

Yes, indeed, Saskatchewan had led the entire world!

EPILOGUE

First universal medicare in North America, 1962
Medicare became law in Saskatchewan on 1 July 1962. However, with inadequate communication and bad timing on both sides, confrontation led to an action not contemplated by the government: withdrawal of services by the great majority of doctors. Each side, government and medical profession, "was convinced of the legitimacy of its role, the rightness of its goals, and of its power to achieve them."[1] Under the distinguished arbitration of Lord Stephen Taylor, a socialist and a medical doctor, who shuttled back and forth between the government and representatives of the Saskatchewan College of Physicians and Surgeons, and earned the trust of both sides, the Saskatoon Agreement was signed on 23 July. The most objective account of this trying time is provided in chapter 5 of Malcolm Taylor's 1978 book.[2]

Why did Saskatchewan take the lead?
Medicare got its start in Saskatchewan because, as in the biblical parable, the seeds fell on fertile ground. The thinly populated, relatively poor province of Saskatchewan consistently led all of Canada in public health innovations and legislation, including twenty-nine firsts. Many of these were firsts for North America, not merely Canada. Even more remarkable were the two instances in which Saskatchewan led the entire world: in the use of the betatron and cobalt-60 to treat cancer. Together, these "building blocks" led logically and sequentially to the first province-wide hospital plan (1947) and the first province-wide medicare plan (1962). But why Saskatchewan?

In a province without a large city, there were few rich people or powerful corporations. Rarely did people have surplus cash, but there was an abundance of good will, of trust in one another, of a willingness to help each other, and of a sense that lives could be improved through communal effort. This was manifest not only in health concerns, but also in the development of the farmer-owned and -operated Saskatchewan Wheat Pool. Mutual co-operation among pioneer settlers was more the rule than the exception; it was better to do things together than separately. If a family had to build a barn, neighbours came to help raise the rafters. The entire community would turn out to build a curling rink.

Saskatchewan residents had a strong sense of justice and fairness. Honesty was the rule. A high priority was given to health matters by the public, especially by farm women. Saskatoon provided an outstanding example when, in 1914, to combat the spread of bovine tuberculosis through milk, it became the first city in the British Empire to forbid the sale of raw milk.

I suggest that the co-operative spirit of the predominantly rural Saskatchewan people, most of them immigrants from Europe, had been developed to a higher and more practical degree than in any other jurisdiction in North America.

The advances made in Saskatchewan required two ingredients: the co-operative spirit, as described above, and the individuals whose passion and direction became the catalyst. It is my thesis that without the unique community spirit, coupled with "the right person in the right place at the right time," some or most of the events recounted here would not have come to pass. These leaders possessed unusual wisdom and prudence. Survivors of the depression, severe drought, and dust storms ("the Dirty Thirties"), these men and women were more frugal than any group since and not in the least litigious. Much effort went unpaid. Every dollar went a long way. The people of Saskatchewan were, to use today's term, proactive. Whether bureaucrat, politician, or scientist, each leader saw a need, gathered the evidence necessary for an informed decision, and then acted expeditiously. Nearly immediate response by government was then more the rule than the exception. Lacking were interminable studies that gathered dust on a shelf. The five most important visionaries were Seymour, Ferguson, Blair, Johns, and Douglas, but others have also played major roles and deserve to be remembered. Each one's effort added to the foundation built by a predecessor. These were simple times, without red tape. The time was right.

Medicare in other provinces

The national initiative of Prime Minister John G. Diefenbaker, the member of parliament from Prince Albert, Saskatchewan, prepared the way for medicare in the rest of Canada. Diefenbaker appointed Mr Justice Emmett M. Hall, chief justice of Saskatchewan to chair a six-member commission. The other six members were not appointed until July 1961.[3] The report was released on 19 June 1964. The report recommended that "as a nation, we now take the necessary … decisions to make all the fruits of the health sciences available to all our residents without hindrance of any kind."[4]

The medicare bill was not passed by the federal government until 16 December 1966. Federal medical care insurance program funding did not become available until 1 July 1968, the date on which the second province, British Columbia, joined. Manitoba, Newfoundland, and Nova Scotia joined in on 1 April 1969; Alberta on 1 July 1969; Ontario on 1 October 1969; Quebec, 1 November 1970; Prince Edward Island, 1 December 1970; New Brunswick, 1 January 1971; and North-West Territories and Yukon on 1 April 1972.[5]

Thus it took almost nine years for medicare to reach all of Canada. Saskatchewan had led, not only in many steps on the road to medicare, but in the implementation of medicare itself.

From a historical perspective, one can look back over the Saskatchewan events chronicled in this book and at least dream about returning to our roots. At the local level, think of the grassroots empowerment felt by the pioneers whose municipal taxes paid for innovative municipal doctors and hospital plans and contributed directly to tuberculosis control and the Swift Current Health Plan!

The loss of local control was brought home to me on 5 July 2002 when I was the guest speaker at the 100th anniversary of the Yorkton hospital. This hospital had a superb nursing training program from 1903 until 1969[6]; the near-overflow crowd at the banquet was composed mainly of nurses who had trained in Yorkton and had gathered from across western Canada to demonstrate their undiminished loyalty and esprit de corps.[7] They still resent the closure of this successful program by centralists. Canada's present nursing shortage (and the doctor shortage in rural areas!) were the predictable result of bad decisions and poor planning that were not evidence-based. Nurses have always been the backbone of the health care system.

Provincially, consider the assumption by both Sigerist and Douglas that the medical school should be the linchpin of the health care system; the unstated corollary would be that it requires commensurate funding. As my father warned T.C. Douglas in 1946, medical schools are extremely expensive and a second-rate medical school would be worse than no medical school.[8] Federally, funding of medicare would be less of a problem if the federal contribution were restored to the 50% provided to each province in the early years, rather than the current figure, said to be about 14%.

Moving medicare forward may ask of us all, at each level, to learn from our history. Can we emulate the co-operative spirit, altruism, and ingenuity shown by Saskatchewan pioneers?

NOTES

Introduction

1 Louis Horlick, "Medicare and Canadian Federalism." In A.M. Herzberg and I. Krupka, eds., *Statistics, Science and Public Policy. The Two Cultures?* Proceedings of the Fourth Conference on Statistics, Science and Public Policy, Hailsham, UK, 1999 (Kingston: Queen's University 1999), 153–8.

2 Eleanor McKinnon. "Open Door Policy." In Ed and Pemrose Whelan, *Touched by Tommy* (Regina: Whelan Publications, 1990), 25.

3 Soon after his interview with Blair and Johns, on 14 November 1949 Douglas turned over the ministry of health to T.J. Bentley, the member from Gull Lake. It was probably more than simple coincidence that Bentley, a farmer, and later on the field staff of the Saskatchewan Wheat Pool, represented a riding within the Swift Current Health Plan.

Chapter One

1 Sally Clubb, *Our Story: 75 Years of Caring* (Saskatoon: St Paul's Hospital, 1982), 2; Marguerite E. Robinson, *The First Fifty Years* (Regina: Saskatchewan Registered Nurses Association, 1967), 8.

2 John Murray Gibbon and Mary S. Mathewson, *Three Centuries of Canadian Nursing* (Toronto: Macmillan, 1947), 214. Not until 1927 was a two-storey brick building, St Joseph's Hospital, built at Ile-à-la-Crosse with government support.

3 H.C. Jamieson, *Early Medicine in Alberta* (Edmonton: Douglas, 1947), 21.

4 R.B. Deane, "Augustus L. Jukes, a Pioneer Surgeon," *Calgary Associate Clinic Historical Bulletin* 2, no. 4 (1938): 1–4.

5 Robinson, *The First Fifty Years*, 8.

6 Joyce Morgan and Barb Straker, "Medical History of Saltcoats." In *Saltcoats Roots and Branches* (Saltcoats: Saltcoats and District Historical Society, 1982), 217–23.

7 At first, residents of Medicine Hat could obtain prepaid hospital insurance at $5 per family per year (Robert Lampard, "Medicare: An Alberta Legacy," *Legacy*, May–July 1998: 34).

8 Lewis Thomas, "Early Territorial Hospitals," *Saskatchewan History* 2, no. 2 (1949): 16–20. In the 1891 census the entire Medicine Hat district had a population of only 1,316. The Calgary hospital opened later in 1890 and the Lethbridge hospital in 1894.

9 Gibbon and Mathewson, *Three Centuries*, 208.

10 In 1901 there were 91,279 people in the area that was to become Saskatchewan in 1905.

11 Personal copies of this large book, owned by each midwifery student in most countries, were affectionately called "Maggie."

12 Robinson, *The First Fifty Years*, 32, 39.
13 Saskatchewan Department of Agriculture, *Annual Report 1906* (Regina), 156–8.
14 A. Becker, "The Lake Geneva Mission, Wakaw, Saskatchewan," *Saskatchewan History* 29 (1976): 51–64.
15 Clubb, *Our Story*, 6.
16 *Saskatoon City Hospital Golden Anniversary, 1909–1959.* (Saskatoon: City Hospital, 1959), 18.
17 Sister Yvonne Bezaire, *Our Roots: A Promise* (Saskatoon: Catholic Health Association of Saskatchewan, 1993), 4.
18 C.S. Houston, "Early Saskatchewan Hospitals," *Annals of the Royal College of Physicians and Surgeons of Canada* 23 (1990): 265–70.

Chapter Two
1 C.S. Houston, "Maurice MacDonald Seymour: A Leader in Public Health," *Annals of the Royal College of Physicians and Surgeons of Canada* 31 (©1998): 41–3, by permission.
2 M.M. Seymour, "Public Health Work in Saskatchewan," *Canadian Medical Association Journal* 15 (1925): 276.
3 Duane John Mombourquette, "A Government and Health Care: The Co-operative Commonwealth Federation in Saskatchewan, 1944–1964" (Master's thesis, University of Regina, 1990), 6.
4 Seymour, *Public Health*, 274.
5 Ibid., 275.
6 Ibid., 277.
7 M.M. Seymour, "A Study of Milk Problems in Canada," *[Canadian] Public Health Journal* 17 (1926a): 241–4; 295–301, 353–8; 394–404.
8 Ibid., 300.
9 M.M. Seymour, "The Seymour Plan," *[Canadian] Public Health Journal* 17 (1926b): 593–6.

10 Seymour, *Public Health*, 275, 277. The Saskatchewan Department of Health *Annual Report* (1929: 95), again made the claim that Saskatchewan was acknowledged as still having the "lowest death rate in the Dominion and in the Empire." Presumably the relative youth of newcomers was the main explanation.

11 Lillian Chase, "Maurice MacDonald Seymour," *Canadian Medical Association Journal* 30 (1929): 212–13.

Chapter Three

1 Duane John Mombourquette, "A Government and Health Care: The Co-operative Commonwealth Federation in Saskatchewan, 1944–1964" (Master's thesis, University of Regina, 1990), 16.

2 Holdfast History and Heritage Committee, *Holdfast, History and Heritage*, 1980, 39.

3 Doris Hungle, "Medical Services." In *Holdfast, History and Heritage*, 83–5. Dilke was the nearest village on the Regina side of Holdfast.

4 A vacancy was pending at Craik, about twenty miles west; the doctor there was about to enlist, and hoped that Schmitt could replace him (Mrs. J.A. Dunn, "Our First Municipal Doctor," *Western Producer*, 1 March 1962).

5 In the 1916 census, the population of Holdfast was 167, Chamberlain 138, Dilke 93, and Penzance 60. Initially, none of the inhabitants of the four villages was covered by the doctor plan. The rural population in RM Sarnia numbered 2,090; taxes earned medical care from Dr Schmitt.

6 C.S. Houston, "Saskatchewan's Municipal Doctors: A Forerunner of the Medicare System that Developed 50 Years Later," *Canadian Medical Association Journal* 151 (1994): 1642–4, by permission.

7 Holdfast History, *Holdfast*, 83.

8 Arthur E. Childe was the municipal doctor for RM Victory #226 at Beechy. Present for only two years, he was nevertheless remembered fondly thirty years later. He became Winnipeg's foremost scientific radiologist, with special skills in pediatric radiology (my field) and neuro-radiology.

9 D.S. Johnstone, "Report of the Committee re Municipal Physicians," *Canadian Medical Association Journal* 17 (1927): xii–xiv.

10 C. Rufus Rorem, *The "Municipal Doctor" System in Rural Saskatchewan* (Chicago: University of Chicago Press, 1931).

11 Ibid., 13. Rorem came to Saskatchewan because of information that Alberta had only two municipal doctors and Manitoba, three.

12 They operated under the provincial Rural Municipality Act of 1929, Sections 168 and 169.

13 Rorem, *"Municipal Doctor,"* 12, 16.

14 Gordon Ferguson, "Income Tax and the Municipal Physician," *Saskatchewan Medical Quarterly* 14, no. 2 (1950): 407–10.

15 Rorem, *"Municipal Doctor,"* 61.

16 Ibid., 62–3.

17 Ibid., 61.

18 Ibid., 74.

19 W.W. Wheeler, "Where Doctors Send No Bills," *Reader's Digest*, July 1935: 75–7.

20 Rorem, *"Municipal Doctor,"* 83–4.

21 G.E. Britnell, "Saskatchewan," *Encyclopedia Canadiana* 9 (1958): 205–28.

22 Mombourquette, "A Government and Health Care," 28–30.

23 Gordon Lawson, "The Co-operative Commonwealth Federation, Health Care Reform, and Physician Remuneration in the Province of Saskatchewan, 1915–1949" (Master's thesis, University of Regina, 1998), 38.

24 R.G. Ferguson, "Report of [the] Committee on Economics,"

Saskatchewan Medical Quarterly 2, no. 4 (1938): 12–18.

25 Ibid., 15.

26 J.J. Collins, "Report of the Municipal Doctors' Question-naire," *Saskatchewan Medical Quarterly* 5, no. 4 (1941): 11–24.

27 Health Services Board, Saskatchewan Medical Association, "Model Municipal Contract," *Saskatchewan Medical Quarterly* 6, no. 2 (1942): 17–25.

28 Lawson, *Co-operative Commonwealth*, 131, 145.

29 Joan Feather and Vincent L. Matthews, "Early Medical Care in Saskatchewan," *Saskatchewan History* 37 (1984): 41–54.

30 Ibid., 47. The ten UHDS were at Davidson, Edam, Eston, Kerrobert, Kindersley, Lloydminster, Lampman, Rosetown, Shaunavon, and Wadena.

31 Statutes of Saskatchewan, 1916, C.12; 1917, C.9; Malcolm G. Taylor, *Health Insurance and Canadian Public Policy*, (Montreal: McGill-Queen's University Press, 1978), 71.

32 A.G. MacKay, *Municipal Hospitals 1919* (Edmonton: Municipal Hospital Branch, 1919).

33 Arthur K. Whiston, *Municipal Hospitals* (Edmonton: Hospitals Branch, Department of Public Health, 1922).

34 Later, in 1948, hospital construction was further supported by federal funds from the National Health Grants Programme, the first federal initiative in health care.

35 F.D. Mott, "Hospital Services in Saskatchewan," *American Journal of Public Health* 37 (1947): 1539–44.

36 Feather and Matthews, "Early Medical Care," 47.

37 Statutes of Saskatchewan: 1918–19, C.100, Section 2. The two rural municipalities named in the Saskatchewan legislation, of course, are both within Saskatchewan; Taylor, *Health Insurance*, 72.

38 Statutes of Saskatchewan: 1927, C.67, The Union Hospital Act, Section 2; 1936, C.37, The Village Act, Section 236; 1936, C.36, The Town Act, Section 8.

39 Malcolm G. Taylor, "The Saskatchewan Hospital Services Plan" (PhD dissertation, University of California, Berkeley, 1949, mimeographed); Taylor, *Health Insurance*, 72.

40 Taylor, *Health Insurance*, 72.

41 Robin F. Badgley and Samuel Wolfe, *Doctors' Strike: Medical Care and Conflict in Saskatchewan* (Toronto: Macmillan, 1967), 24.

42 Saskatchewan Statutes 1934–35, C.30, Section 245.

43 Taylor, *Health Insurance*, 72.

Chapter Four

1 C.S. Houston, *R.G. Ferguson, Crusader Against Tuberculosis* (Toronto: Hannah Institute and Dundurn Press, 1991), by permission Associated Medical Services Inc. through its Hannah Institute for the History of Medicine Program.

2 A.B. Cook, R.G. Ferguson, J.F. Cairns, and R.H. Brighton, *Report of the Saskatchewan Anti-tuberculosis Commission* (Regina: J.W. Reid, King's Printer, 1922).

3 Helen Ferguson, "That a Child Might Live," *Valley Echo* 40, no. 12 (1959): 4–6.

4 H. Boughton, "A.C.T. Million Dollar Story," *Valley Echo* 45, no. 3 (1964): 19–20.

5 Saskatchewan Anti-tuberculosis League. *Annual Report,* 1942.

6 Conveying formal membership in the prestigious Royal College of Physicians, thus allowing use of the initials MRCP.

7 Houston, *R.G. Ferguson,* 58.

8 Cook et al., *Report ... Anti-tuberculosis Commission.*

9 R.G. Ferguson, "A Tuberculosis Survey of 1,346 School Children in Saskatchewan," *Canadian Medical Association Journal* 12 (1922): 381–3.

10 G.J. Wherrett, *The Miracle of the Empty Beds: A History of Tuberculosis in Canada* (Toronto: University of Toronto Press, 1977), 35, 187. In 1922, the Canadian Red Cross provided funds for the Canadian Tuberculosis Association to undertake similar representative school surveys in the other provinces.

11 G.J. Wherrett and S. Grzybowski, *Report and Recommendations on Tuberculosis Control in Saskatchewan* (Ottawa: Department of National Health and Welfare, 1966), 8.

12 Jean B.D. Larmour, *A Matter of Life and Breath: The 75-year History of the Saskatchewan Anti-tuberculosis League and the Saskatchewan Lung Association* (Saskatoon: Saskatchewan Lung Association, 1987), 18, augmented by Dr Dudley G. Barnett, personal communication, May 2002.

13 Houston, *R.G. Ferguson*, 81–2.

14 Ibid., 83.

15 Wherrett & Grzybowski, "Report and Recommendations," 5,6

16 Houston, *R.G. Ferguson, Ibid.*, 83.

17 Ibid., 84.

18 R.G. Ferguson, "Tuberculosis Among the Indians of the Great Canadian Plains," *Transactions of the National Association for the Prevention of Tuberculosis* 14 (1928): 625–45.

19 C.S. Houston, "Ferguson's BCG Research: Canada's First Randomized Clinical Trial?" *Investigative Medicine* 16 (1983): 89–91.

20 R.G. Ferguson and A.B. Simes, "BCG Vaccination of Indian Infants in Saskatchewan," *Tubercle* 30 (1949): 5–11.

21 R.G. Ferguson, "BCG Vaccination in Hospitals and Sanatoria

of Saskatchewan," *Canadian Journal of Public Health* 37 (1946): 435–51.

22 G.D. Barnett, "Results of Mass Surveys in the Province of Saskatchewan, 1942–1947," *Canadian Tuberculosis Association Annual Papers* 50 (1950): 33–6.

23 Wherrett, *Miracle*, 255. Later, from 1941 through 1955, Ontario had the lowest TB death rate, except for 1944 and 1954, when Saskatchewan briefly regained the lead.

24 Anonymous, *Canadian Tuberculosis Association Bulletin* 22, no. 2 (1943): 4; Wherrett and Grzybowski, *Report and Recommendations*, 7–8.

25 Wherrett and Grzybowski, *Report and Recommendations*, 4. In Canada, only the Manitoba Sanatorium Board was similarly constituted.

26 Ibid., 10.

27 Larmour, *A Matter of Life*, 101–15.

28 R.G. Ferguson, *Studies in Tuberculosis* (Toronto: University of Toronto Press, 1955).

29 C. Smith, "Saskatchewan's 'Health Hero' Enshrined in Hearts of People." *Saskatchewan Health Newsletter* 15, no. 3 (1964): 2,15.

30 V.H. Hoeppner, *Life and Breath* 1, no. 3 (August 1989): 4.

31 Houston, *R.G. Ferguson*, 134–6.

32 V.H. Hoeppner "Tuberculosis in Saskatchewan Treaty Indians," *Prairie Medical Journal* 65 (1995): 18–20.

33 Ibid., 19–20.

Chapter Five

1 E.W. Barootes, "The Role of Saskatchewan in Government-Sponsored Health Care: A Retrospective Review," *Annals of the Royal College of Physicians and Surgeons of Canada* 24, 2 (1991): 117–19.

2 Thomas H. McLeod and Ian McLeod, *Tommy Douglas: The Road to Jerusalem* (Edmonton: Hurtig, 1987), 112. This is a superb biography of Douglas.

3 During its final fifteen months in office, W.J. Patterson's Liberal government had appointed two committees to study the possibility of health insurance. The bipartisan Select Special Committee of 25 Liberal and CCF MLAS, chaired by Bamm Hogarth, a Liberal MLA from Regina, had been appointed on 2 March 1943; they gave an interim report on 12 April 1943 and a final report on 31 March 1944. The Saskatchewan Reconstruction Council, established on 20 October 1943, did not give its final report until August 1944, after the election. Sigerist made "extensive use" of the briefs presented to both groups (Gordon S. Lawson, "The Co-operative Commonwealth Federation, Health Reform and Physician Remuneration in the Province of Saskatchewan, 1915–1949" [Master's thesis, University of Regina, 1998], 50–4).

4 Dr Hugh MacLean, a Regina surgeon from 1913 to 1938, and CCF candidate in the 1935 federal election, advised Douglas to take the health portfolio (Jacalyn Duffin, "The Guru and the Godfather: Henry Sigerist, Hugh MacLean, and the Politics of Health Care Reform in 1940s Canada," *Canadian Bulletin of Medical History* 9 [1992]: 191–218).

5 Douglas phoned Sigerist first on 16 June. (Nora Sigerist Beeson, *Henry E. Sigerist: Autobiographical Writings* [Montreal: McGill University Press, 1966], 187).

6 Henry E. Sigerist, *Socialized Medicine in the Soviet Union* (New York: W.W. Norton, 1937).

7 Malcolm G. Taylor, *Health Insurance and Canadian Public Policy* (Montreal: McGill-Queen's University Press, 1978), 88, 434.

8 Also assisting Sigerist were Dr Mindel Cherniak Sheps, a family practitioner and Manitoba CCF executive member from Winnipeg, as secretary; Ann Heffel, a nurse; C.C. Gibson, a hospital administrator; and Dr J.L. Connell, a dentist. (Mombourquette, "A Government and Health Care: the Co-operative Commonwealth Federation in Saskatchewan, 1944–64" [Master's thesis, University of Regina, 1990], 54.)

9 Beeson, *Henry E. Sigerist*, 190.

10 H.E. Sigerist, *Report of the Commissioner* (Regina: Health Services Survey Commission, 1944).

11 Ibid., 5.

12 This figure was unrealistic, given that the average cost of hospitalization per capita in Saskatchewan had that year already reached $5.20, having risen from $1.93 in 1934 (Malcolm G. Taylor, "The Saskatchewan Hospital Services Plan" [PhD dissertation, University of California, Berkeley, 1949, mimeographed], 140.)

13 Sigerist, *Report of the Commissioner*, 5.

14 Cited by Taylor, *Health Insurance*, 434.

15 Beeson, *Henry E. Sigerist*, 231.

16 Lawson's 1998 thesis explains how fee-for-service payment became entrenched, and why the CCF government chose not to follow the Health Services Planning Commission's recommendation that doctors be placed on salary.

17 T.C. Douglas to Dr J.L. Brown, letter reprinted in *Saskatchewan Medical Quarterly* 9, no. 3 (1945): 31–4.

18 Taylor, *Health Insurance*, 87.

19 Advisory Committee on Health Insurance, *Report* (Ottawa: 1942–43). This 558-page report was presented by Chairman J.J. Heagerty to the House of Commons in December 1942.

20 Taylor, *Health Insurance*, 252.

21 To achieve this, the doctors agreed to a fixed sum of money for any given year.

22 Taylor, *Health Insurance*, 244.

23 The social assistance plan was administered by the Medical Services Division of the Saskatchewan Department of Public Health (Ibid., 252).

24 Ibid., 252.

25 Mombourquette, *A Government and Health Care*, 119.

26 McLeod and McLeod, *Tommy Douglas*, 312.

Chapter Six

1 Joan Feather, "From Concept to Reality: Formation of the Swift Current Health Region," *Prairie Forum* 16 (1991a): 59.

2 Hazlet Historical Society, *Hazlet and Its Heritage* (Hazlet 1987), 1:3.

3 Somewhat similar plans which, unlike the municipal doctor plans, allowed free choice of doctor, had begun in Alberta at Cardston in 1932 (Beryl Shaw, "Medicare in Cardston." In *Chief Mountain Country: A History of Cardston and District*. [Cardston: Cardston and District Historical Society, 1987], 72–4), and at Lamont in 1933 where, for the first two years, "services exceeded payment five-fold." (Robert Lampard, "Medicare: An Alberta Legacy," *Legacy*, May-July 1948: 34–5). The Cardston plan ran until 1968; Shaw failed to claim this as "the longest continuously run (thirty-six years) prepaid community based medical insurance program in Canada." (Robert Lampard, unpublished ms.).

4 Feather, "From Concept to Reality," 70.

5 Syd Munt, "How the Swift Current Region Was Organized." (Mimeographed, 3 pages, 1946). As postmaster at Hazlet, Munt had handled the voluminous mail sent out by Burak the previous year.

6 Webb History Book Committee, *Prairie Memories* (Webb, 1982), 62.

7 *Swift Current Sun*, 25 August 1945.

8 Munt, "How the Swift Current Region," 1.

9 Lester Jorgenson, "Rural Municipality of Miry Creek No. 229 and Health Region No. 1." In *Bridging the Centuries* (Abbey, SK: Miry Creek Area History Book Committee, 2000), 52–8.

10 F.D. Mott, "Prepaid Medical Care under Governmental Auspices in Saskatchewan," *Canadian Journal of Public Health* 41 (1950): 403–10.

11 Munt, "How the Swift Current Region," 1. Burak met in person with Dave Belbeck of the *Swift Current Sun*, S.H. Gamble of the *Gull Lake Advance*, and W. Sharpe of the *Shaunavon Standard*.

12 Burak attended council meetings at RM Grassy Creek #78 at Shaunavon, RM Arlington #79 at Dollard, RM Bone Creek #108 at Instow, RM Carmichael #109, and RM Gull Lake #139.

13 Feather, "From Concept to Reality," 72–3.

14 Ibid., 74.

15 T.C. Douglas, "The Doctor in Saskatchewan's Health Plans," *Saskatchewan Medical Quarterly* 9, no. 1 (1945): 24–31.

16 Feather, "From Concept to Reality," 74.

17 Munt, "How the Swift Current Region," 2.

18 Burak suffered a personal disappointment. Stewart Robertson was appointed to the job that he had coveted. Burak moved to become secretary-treasurer in other municipalities at Hafford, Ogema, and lastly RM Aberdeen #373. He died in Saskatoon on 8 June 1976.

19 Feather, "From Concept to Reality," 74.

20 Pat Cammer, "Some Memories of the Beginnings of Health Region #1" (Typescript of speech given at the final Swift Current Health Region information meeting, Swift Current, 3 June 1993).

21 Feather, "From Concept to Reality," 75.

22 Sadly, on 5 December 2001, a Health bureaucrat in Regina, lacking any sense of history or justice, renumbered Saskatchewan's health regions, from east to west. Swift Current was stripped of its historical right to continue a hallowed tradition as "Number One" not only in Saskatchewan, but Number One in all North America.

23 Stewart Robertson, "New Horizons for Better Health." *In Winds of Change* (Swift Current: Swift Current Health Region, 1966), 23–6. From the beginning the plan provided a dental program for children.

24 The vice-president was Ken Rutherford, a school principal who was also mayor of Swift Current. In 1960, Ken was an unsuccessful CCF candidate in the 1960 provincial election in British Columbia.

25 Drs O.M. Irwin and R.R. Stirrett of Swift Current, Dr J.A. Matheson of Gull Lake, and Dr F.B. Dawson of Maple Creek.

26 Dr Lloyd Davey lasted only five months. Later, Peart was general secretary of the Canadian Medical Association, based in Toronto in 1966.

27 Dr Alan Gregg of the Rockefeller Foundation, when touring western Canada to examine medical services, visited the Health Services Planning Commission in Regina. In answer to the question, "In which countries are health services supplied to residents ... under a plan sponsored by the State," he answered: 1. Russia. 2. Peping [Beijing] China, for 200,000 people. 3. Swift Current Health Region No. 1. This

story was related to the first annual meeting of Health Region No. 1 on 25 September 1947 by Carl Kjorven.

28 Apart from one leave, when he still served part-time.

29 Fred D. Mott, "Prepaid Medical Care," 403–10. Mott called this unique arrangement a "dual and yet co-ordinated program of community and personal health services."

30 Vince Matthews was director, Medical and Hospital Services Branch, 1957–62; acting deputy minister, 1962–63; and associate deputy minister, 1963–64, Saskatchewan Department of Health. Thereafter he was professor and head, Department of Social and Preventive Medicine at the University of Saskatchewan. He retired as professor emeritus in 1987 and died suddenly on 7 October 1988.

31 Swift Current Health Region, *Winds of Change*, 8.

32 Two surgeons, an obstetrician and an anaesthetist.

33 J. Lloyd Brown, "Swift Current Health Insurance Scheme," *Saskatchewan Medical Quarterly* 13 (1949): 251–8.

34 Cammer, "Some Memories." In April 1947, when she married Ross Cammer, a farmer west of Webb, Patricia Ditner left her position as Stewart Robertson's secretary.

35 Dr Orville Hjertaas, interview by Maureen Matthews, "The Origins of Medicare," *Ideas*, Canadian Broadcasting Corporation, 5 December 1990, transcript, 2.

36 Cammer, "Some Memories."

37 Brown, "Swift Current Health Insurance," 254.

38 J.A. Matheson, O.M. Irwin, F.R. Dawson, and G.G. Ferguson, "Report of the Swift Current Health Region No. 1," *Saskatchewan Medical Quarterly* 11 (1947): 21–5.

39 Ibid., 24.

40 Brown, "Swift Current Health Insurance," 255.

41 J.A. Matheson, "Swift Current Health Service," *Saskatchewan Medical Quarterly* 14 (1950): 368–70.

42 Gordon Howden, "General Practice in Health Region No. 1," *Saskatchewan Medical Quarterly* 13 (1949): 335–9.

43 Swift Current Health Region, *Winds of Change*, 55.

44 A.D. Kelly, "The Swift Current Experiment," *Canadian Medical Association Journal* 58 (1946): 506–511.

45 V.L. Matthews, "Patterns for Progress Emerge." In Swift Current Health Region, *Winds of Change*, 18–21.

46 Maureen is the daughter of the late Dr Vincent L. Matthews.

47 Maureen Matthews, "The Origins of Medicare," *Ideas*, Canadian Broadcasting Corporation, 5 December 1990, transcript, 10.

48 Ibid., 5, 8.

49 Jorgenson, "Rural Municipality of Miry Creek," 56.

50 Ibid.

51 Joan Feather, "Impact of the Swift Current Health Region: Experiment or Model?" *Prairie Forum* 16 (1991b): 225–48.

52 Swift Current Health Region, "The Swift Current Medical – Dental Program, 1946 to 1962." (Mimeographed, n.d.).

53 Feather, "Impact," 243.

54 Jorgenson, "Rural Municipality of Miry Creek," 57.

55 Malcolm G. Taylor, *Health Insurance and Canadian Public Policy* (Montreal: McGill-Queen's University Press, 1978), 266.

56 Vince Matthews (Address to annual meeting, Swift Current Health Region Board, 5 June 1985).

57 I was shocked to realize that Saskatchewan lagged behind other provinces in establishing rural health regions. The Swift Current Health Region No. 1 was the only fully functioning health region in Saskatchewan – in one respect a beacon in a land of darkness; by 1943, all other provinces except Saskatchewan had a system of rural public health

units for preventive medicine (Feather, "From Concept to Reality," 66).

58 Jorgenson, "Rural Municipality of Miry Creek," 55.

Chapter Seven

1 There had been a two-year basic science medical course in the School of Medicine at the University of Saskatchewan since 1926. Students then went to Alberta, Manitoba or Ontario to take their clinical years of instruction.

2 Henry E. Sigerist, *Report of the Commissioner* (Regina: Health Services Survey Commission, 1944), 11.

3 Gibson went on to become professor of neurological research and of the history of medicine at the University of British Columbia.

4 Douglas J. Buchan, *Greenhouse to Medical Centre: Saskatchewan's Medical School 1926–1978* (Saskatoon: University of Saskatchewan, 1983), 39.

5 On a personal note, my medical class at the University of Manitoba elected Wendell Macleod as our honourary president. As a result, he gave the address, "The Gold-headed Cane" at our graduating banquet in Winnipeg in 1951.

6 Buchan, *Greenhouse*, 21–2.

7 Ibid.

8 Louis Horlick, *Medical College to Community Resource: Saskatchewan's Medical School, 1978–1998* (Saskatoon: University of Saskatchewan, 1999).

9 Louis Horlick, *They Built Better Than They Knew: Saskatchewan's Royal University Hospital. A History, 1955–1992* (Saskatoon: Royal University Hospital Foundation, 2001), 16.

10 Ibid., 19.

11 Buchan, *Greenhouse*, 36.
12 Horlick, *They Built Better*.

Chapter Eight

1 W. Douglas Piercey, "Hospitals," *Encyclopedia Canadiana* 5 (1958): 161–4.
2 Duane John Mombourquette, "A Government and Health Care: The Co-operative Commonwealth Federation in Saskatchewan." (Master's thesis, University of Regina, 1990), 68.
3 Ibid., 103–4.
4 H.E. Sigerist, *Report of the Commissioner* (Regina: Health Services Survey Commission, 1944), 7.
5 Aided by "provincial hospital construction grants ... the ratio of hospital beds to population increased from 4.8 per 1,000 in 1946 to 6.5 per 1,000 in 1951." (Malcolm G. Taylor, *Health Insurance and Canadian Public Policy* [Montreal: McGill-Queen's University Press, 1978], 103–4).
6 Louis Horlick, *They Built Better Than They Knew: Saskatchewan's Royal University Hospital. A History, 1995–1992* (Saskatoon: Royal University Hospital Foundation, 2001), 10.
7 Most doctors were also accepting of Thomas H. McLeod, the brilliant economist seconded to the Health Services Planning Commission, but they were suspicious of Dr Cecil Sheps, Mott's predecessor, and especially of Cecil's wife, Mindel, who had served for a longer time as secretary of the HSPC. Most medical doctors thought this couple had too much power, and sensed that they wished to impose their version of socialist ideology on the province.
8 Taylor, *Health Insurance*, 102–3.
9 Hospitals were graded and paid a per diem rate that varied with the facilities and services provided (Ibid., 102).

10 Ibid., 103.

11 F.D. Mott, "Prepaid Medical Care under Government Auspices in Saskatchewan," *Canadian Journal of Public Health* 41 (1950), 407.

12 F.D. Mott, "Hospital Services in Saskatchewan," *American Journal of Public Health* 37 (1947): 1542.

13 Taylor, *Health Insurance*, 104, 435.

14 Milton I. Roemer, "'Socialized' Health Services in Saskatchewan," *Social Research* 25 (1958): 87–101.

15 Privy Council (Canada) 3408. This was followed by Saskatchewan Order-in-Council 74/49 on 11 January 1949.

16 By chance, two other members in addition to my father, Dr C.J. Houston, were from Yorkton, population 5,000. City clerk Howard Jackson represented the Saskatchewan Urban Municipalities Association and newspaper publisher S.N. Wynn represented the Saskatchewan Hospital Association.

17 C.S. Houston, "The Early Years of the *Saskatchewan Medical Quarterly*," *Canadian Medical Association Journal* 118 (1978): 118–19, by permission.

18 Ken McTaggart, *The First Decade* (Ottawa: Canadian Medical Association, 1973), 43.

19 C.J. Houston, "Report," *Saskatchewan Medical Quarterly* 15, no. 4 (1951), 626.

20 Health Survey Committee, *Saskatchewan Health Survey Report* (Regina: Government of Saskatchewan, 1951), 225. During these meetings, Malcolm Taylor and C.J. Houston became lifelong friends. Taylor later was in charge of research for the federal Royal Commission on Health Services chaired by Saskatchewan Chief Justice Emmett Hall, 1961–64.

21 Taylor, *Health Insurance*, 233.

Chapter Nine

1 Fannie H. Kahan, *Brains and Bricks: The History of the Yorkton Psychiatric Centre* (Regina: White Cross Publications, 1965), 13–15.

2 Ibid., 16.

3 Harley Dickinson, *The Two Psychiatries: The Transformation of Psychiatric Work in Saskatchewan, 1905–1984* (Regina: Canadian Plains Research Centre, 1989), 21.

4 Colin M. Smith, "Mental Health Services in Saskatchewan, 1914–1978" (Typescript of talk given to psychiatry rounds, University Hospital, 17 February 1984).

5 Colin M. Smith, "A Decade of Psychiatry in Saskatchewan," *Saskatchewan Medical Quarterly* 38, no. 3 (1974): 31–3.

6 Humphrey Osmond, quoted in Kahan, *Brains and Bricks*, 25, 83.

7 M.C. Schreder and Colin M. Smith, "La formation des infirmiers psychiatriques," *Information Psychiatrique* 50 (1974): 489–94.

8 Instruction for untrained ward attendants had begun in 1930, but they received only sixty hours of lectures over two years.

9 C.M. Smith and L.L. McKay, "The Open Psychiatric Ward and Its Vicissitudes," *American Journal of Psychiatry* 121 (1965): 763–7.

10 C.M. Smith and D.G. McKerracher, "The Comprehensive Psychiatric Unit in the General Hospital," *American Journal of Psychiatry* 121 (1964): 52–7.

11 D.G. McKerracher, "Psychiatry in General Practice," *Canadian Medical Association Journal* 88 (1963): 1014–16.

12 W.A. Cassell, C.M. Smith, F. Grunberg, J.A. Boan, and R.F. Thomas, "Comparing Costs of Hospital and Community

Care," *Hospital and Community Psychiatry* 23 (1972): 197–200.

13 F.S. Lawson and K. Izumi, "The Saskatchewan Plan," *Mental Hospitals* 8 (1957): 27–31. Dr Ian McDonald informs me that McKerracher was also at the Denver meeting in 1956, but was watching television – a World Series baseball game famous that day for a no-hitter – while Lawson delivered the paper on the Saskatchewan Plan.

14 Mills, a retired psychology professor from the University of Saskatchewan, is researching the Saskatchewan Plan.

15 Kahan, *Brains and Bricks*, 27.

16 Saskatchewan's first and only cottage mental hospital, adjacent to the new 200-bed regional hospital, opened in Yorkton in October 1963, with five cottages of thirty beds each.

17 Smith, "A Decade of Psychiatry," 31.

18 D.G. McKerracher, "Psychiatric Care in Transition," *Mental Hygiene* 45 (1961): 3–9.

19 D.G. McKerracher, Department of Psychiatry, *Annual Report*, 1963. University of Saskatchewan Archives.

20 Ibid.

21 W.J. McCorkell and D.G. McKerracher, "The Family Doctor and the Psychiatric Ward," *Mental Hospitals* 13 (1962): 300–2.

22 The rural equivalent was at Central Butte, where the three family practitioners received regular twice-monthly support from a visiting psychiatrist for two years. (L.W. Christ, E. Christ, and G.W. Mainprize, "Observations on the Psychiatric Project at Central Butte, Saskatchewan," *Canadian Family Physician* 13 [1967]: 35–41).

23 D.G. McKerracher, C.M. Smith, F.E. Coburn, and I.M. McDonald, "General-Practice Psychiatry: Two Canadian Experiments, *Lancet* 2 (1965): 1005–7.

Chapter Ten

1 Ellice had been named for his birthplace, Fort Ellice, the Hudson's Bay Company post on the Manitoba-Saskatchewan boundary.

2 The son of Archibald McDonald, an HBC fur trader, Ellice had graduated in medicine from McGill University with his MB BCH in 1901.

3 Murray to Dunning, 6 October 1922. Premier Dunning papers Y–16–0, pages 25, 918–19 (unpublished letters), Saskatchewan Archives Board (SAB), M6.

4 Dunning to Murray, 11 October 1922, SAB, M6.

5 B.W. Currie, "Ertle Leslie Harrington, 1887-1956," *Proceedings and Transactions of the Royal Society of Canada* 50 (1956): 91.

6 R.O. Davison, "Saskatchewan's Programme for Cancer Control," *Canadian Public Health Journal* 24 (1933): 566–71.

7 A. Becker, "A Sketch of Radiology at St. Paul's Hospital," *Saskatchewan Medical Quarterly* 34 (1970): 34–6.

8 J. Hawkes, *The Story of Saskatchewan and Its People* (Regina: S.J. Clarke, 1924), 1720–1; "Obituary: Dr Clarence Henry," *Canadian Medical Association Journal* 70 (1954): 701.

9 Anonymous, "400 K.V. X-ray Therapy Unit Now Available in This Province," *Saskatchewan Medical Quarterly* 2 (1935): 22.

10 For a "nominal" fee of $10, an appreciable amount in those times (Duane John Mombourquette, "A Government and Health Care: The Co-operative Commonwealth Federation in Saskatchewan, 1944–1964" [Master's thesis, University of Regina, 1990], 25).

11 Charles R. Hayter, "Compromising on Cancer: The Saskatchewan Cancer Commission and the Medical Profession, 1930-1940," *Saskatchewan History* 54 (2002): 5–17.

12 Mombourquette, *A Government and Health Care*, 25.

13 D.V. Cormack, "The Saskatchewan Radon Plant, 1931–1962," *Physics in Canada* 41 (1985): 3–5.

14 Blair had trained as a surgeon in Winnipeg. Following concentrated cancer training at centres in Great Britain, France, Germany, Belgium and Sweden, he was employed as a cancer specialist at New York Memorial Hospital, the University of Alabama, and then the University of Toronto.

15 Contrary to popular belief in Saskatchewan, Alberta offered free cancer treatment in Calgary and Edmonton, beginning in 1941. Saskatchewan was not first in this regard.

16 M.S. Acker and T.A. Watson, "Saskatchewan's Experience with a Comprehensive Public Cancer Program," *American Journal of Public Health* 50 (1960): 65–73.

17 Anonymous, "Portraits in Radiology: Harold Elford Johns, PhD," *Applied Radiology* 1978: 25.

18 Harold Johns,, Transcript of interview by Lauriston S. Taylor, Rockville, Maryland, 17 October 1979, cited in C.S. Houston and S.O. Fedoruk, "Radiation Therapy in Saskatchewan." In J.E. Aldrich and B.C. Lentle, eds., *A New Kind of Ray* (Vancouver: University of British Columbia, 1995), 426.

19 Six years later, in November 1952, the Saskatchewan Division of the Canadian Cancer Society gave Sylvia Fedoruk a $1,000 travelling fellowship to cover a two-month visit to cancer treatment sites in Chicago, Cincinnati, Detroit, New York, Oak Ridge and San Francisco; her expenses came to $996.

20 Houston and Fedoruk, "Radiation Therapy," 147.

21 McNaughton had been born to a pioneer family at Moosomin, 25 February 1887. Trained as an engineer at McGill University, he was president of the Atomic Energy Control Board of Canada, 1946–48.

22 C.S. Houston and S.O. Fedoruk, "Saskatchewan's Role in Radiotherapy Research," *Canadian Medical Association Journal* 132 (©1985): 854–64, by permission.

23 H.E. Johns, "AAPM Coolidge Award," *Medical Physics* 3 (1976): 375.

24 Houston and Fedoruk, "Saskatchewan's Role," 858.

25 E.L. Harrington, R.N.H. Haslam, H.E. Johns, and L. Katz, "The Betatron Building and Installation at the University of Saskatchewan," *Science* 110 (1949): 283–5; H.E. Johns, E.K. Darby, R.N.H. Haslam, L. Katz, and E.L. Harrington, "Depth Dose Data and Isodose Distributions for Radiation from a 22 Mev Betatron," *American Journal of Roentgenology* 62 (1949): 257–68; H.E. Johns, E.K. Darby, and R.O. Kornelson, "The Physical Aspects of Treatment of Cancer by 22 Mev X-rays," *British Journal of Radiology* 24 (1951): 355–64; S.O. Fedoruk, H.E. Johns, and T.A. Watson, "Isodose Distributions for a 1100 Curie Cobalt 60 unit," *Radiology* 60 (1953): 348–54. (Sixteen additional papers concerning radiation dose measurements are cited in Houston and Fedoruk, "Radiation Therapy," 426).

26 M.D. Schulz, "The Supervoltage Story," *American Journal of Roentgenology* 124 (1975): 541–59.

27 Houston and Fedoruk, "Radiation Therapy," 147.

28 Johns, letter to the president, Saskatchewan Division of the Canadian Cancer Society, cited in Houston and Fedoruk, "Saskatchewan's Role," 858.

29 Timing of this visit was perfect. Less than three months later, on 14 November 1949, Douglas gave up the demanding health portfolio, but of course stayed on as premier.

30 Houston and Fedoruk, "Radiation Therapy," 149.

31 Houston and Fedoruk, "Saskatchewan's Role," 859.

32 Sybil Johns, "At Home with the Atom," *Mayfair Magazine* 30 (July 1955): 30–1 and 53–8.

33 Houston and Fedoruk, "Radiation Therapy," 149.

34 Ibid., 149-50.

35 Ibid., 150.

36 Ibid., 151.

37 Date of death obtained from Medical Records, Saskatoon Cancer Agency. A recent article by historian Paul Litt, "Photon Finish: The Race to Build the Bomb," *Beaver* 82, no. 2 (April-May 2002): 28–31, fails to mention the drastic difference in the survival of the first two patients treated, nor does it mention that only one of the cobalt-60 machines had been carefully calibrated.

38 W.C. von Röntgen, "On a New Kind of Ray," *Proceedings of the Physical-Medical Society of Würzburg, 28 December 1895*; second communication 1896. Röntgen could have become a very wealthy man, but he deliberately refrained from taking a patent on his invention; he wished to share it with the world.

39 H.E. Johns, L.M. Bates, E.R. Epp, D.V. Cormack, and S.O. Fedoruk, "1,000-curie Cobalt-60 Units for Radiation Therapy," Nature 168 (1951): 1035–8.

40 A. Morrison, W.R. Dixon, C. Garrett, H.E. Johns, L.M. Bates, E.R. Epp, D.V. Cormack, and S.O. Fedoruk, "Multicurie Cobalt 60 Units for Radiation Therapy," *Science* 115 (1952): 310–12.

41 As isodose curves.

42 D. Cassels, "Brave New Worlds for Nuclear Medicine," *Ascent* 1 (1979): 8-10.

43 Houston and Fedoruk, "Radiation Therapy," 154.

Epilogue

1 Malcolm G. Taylor, *Health Insurance and Canadian Public Policy* (Montreal: McGill-Queen's University Press, 1978), 239–330.

2 Ibid.; E.A. Tollefson, *Bitter Medicine: The Saskatchewan Medicare Feud* (Saskatoon, Modern Press, 1964) provides a legal viewpoint. Robin F. Badgley and Samuel Wolfe, *Doctors' Strike: Medical Care and Conflict in Saskatchewan* (Toronto: Macmillan, 1967) is a third recommended source.

3 Two medical doctors, David M. Baltzan of Saskatoon and Arthur van Wart of Fredericton, New Brunswick; Dean Alice Gerard of the University of Montreal School of Nursing; Dr Leslie Strachan, a dentist from London, Ontario; Wallace McCutcheon, an industrialist from Ontario, and Dr O.J. Firestone, an economist. Dr Malcolm G. Taylor was research consultant and Professor Bernard Blishen was research director.

4 Taylor, *Health Insurance*, 342.

5 Ibid., 375.

6 As a family practitioner in Yorkton, 1951–60, my assigned role was to teach the student nurses about dermatology and sexually transmitted diseases.

7 Fourteen of the twenty-one members of the class of 1962 returned; that evening they sang two songs as part of the entertainment.

8 When the new medical school was about to open in Newfoundland in 1967, and Lord Stephen Taylor was president of Memorial University, I was offered the headship of diagnostic radiology. I have since admired from afar the funding and stability of that department. Free from the intervening level of bureaucracy of a city-wide health board, which in Saskatoon has yet to develop appreciable priorities for either teaching or research, it appears to me that impoverished Newfoundland regards its medical school as a provincial resource and treasure.

INDEX

Unless otherwise specified, towns listed here are in Saskatchewan.

Numbers in italics indicate photos

Index

Index